1982

Health-Care Finance

Health-Care Finance

An Analysis of Cost and Utilization Issues

Robert J. Buchanan
California State College

LexingtonBooks
D.C. Heath and Company
Lexington, Massachusetts
Toronto

Library of Congress Cataloging in Publication Data

Buchanan, Robert John.
  Health-care finance.

  Bibliography: p.
  1. Nursing homes—United States—Finance. 2. Nursing homes—
United States—Rates. 3. Nursing homes, Proprietary—United States—
Finance. 4. Medicaid. [DNLM: 1. Costs and cost analysis. 2. Insurance, Health, Reimbursement. 3. Reimbursement mechanics. 4. Nursing homes. 5. Health insurance for aged and disabled, Title 18. 6. Medical assistance, Title 19. 7. Long term care. 8. Nursing homes—Utilization. WT 30 B918h]
RA997.B79   338.4'336216'0973   80-8362
ISBN 0-669-04035-5

Copyright © 1981 by D.C. Heath and Company.

Published simultaneously in Canada

Printed in the United States of America

International Standard Book Number: 0-669-04035-5

Library of Congress Catalog Card Number: 80-8362

*To my Mother
and
to Liz, Kristin, and Mitchell*

Contents

Contents

List of Tables

Acknowledgments

This book grew out of a health-care grant awarded by the Pharmaceutical Manufacturer's Association. I thank Margaret Zusky, Carolyn Yoder, Kathleen Benn, and the other people at Lexington Books who assisted with the preparation of the book. The comments and advice of Professors Weldon Cooper, Steven Rhoads, and Laurin Henry were helpful in developing the research. Federal and state Medicaid officials and congressional staff personnel also provided needed data for this project. Particularly helpful were Ms. Lily Taylor of the Department of Health and Human Services and Ms. Marilyn Glick, assistant to Congressman Jerry Lewis. Marc Levin of the American Health Care Association provided other needed information. My friends at the Federal Executive Institute were invaluable to the completion of this book. Without their cooperation it would have been far more difficult to gather the data needed for this analysis.

1

Introduction: The Long-Term-Care System

In the United States more than one million people, or one out of every twenty elderly Americans, require a degree of health care that can only be provided by a long-term-care institution.[1] National studies indicate that 8 percent of the American population over age 65 who are living in the community are either completely bedfast or housebound. An additional 6 percent can leave their homes only with assistance.[2] Although not all of these elderly people necessarily require institutional care, these statistics do indicate a large potential base of consumer demand for long-term, health-care-related services. As the percentage of elderly in the American population increases, this demand will become more acute.

The Medicare and Medicaid programs have provided much of the purchasing power to translate this medical need for specialized health care into a market demand. To minimize inefficiency in the delivery of health-care services, and to minimize public-sector health-care costs, we must recognize the unique health needs of the elderly and plan for those health-related services that can satisfy these needs at a minimum cost. Since federal and state governments are the primary purchasers of health-care services for the elderly—60 percent of the $26.68 billion spent in 1974 was from public funds[3]—the public sector has a major responsibility to guarantee the quality of the services consumed, to plan for an adequate supply of these services, and to utilize public resources to maximize social benefit.

The Long-Term-Care Institution

The long-term-care institution, which is a major component of the health-care services needed by the elderly, has a unique role in the total health-delivery system. This role is distinct from the need for the acute-care hospital. To understand this distinction, comparing and contrasting the objectives of these different organizations in treating their respective patients, is useful.

The acute-care, short-term general hospital is organized to treat and cure an acute disease or condition. "It is in fact a disease-oriented facility with its attention directed to the abnormality rather than to the total human configuration."[4]

In contrast, the long-term-care facility has a more-limited range of

1

objectives for its patients. The ideal goal of recovery at the acute-care hospital is replaced by "the more-mundane objective of partial rehabilitation, helping the patient to live within the limitations of his illness, and facilitating his comfort."[5]

The long-term-care facility fills the void in the health-delivery system between the acute-care hospital and the patient's home. After a patient has been diagnosed, treated, and the medical status has been stabilized or cured, the patient is ready for discharge from the acute-care hospital. However, many patients, especially the elderly, may not be ready or able to return to the community. Such persons may need additional physical, emotional, and social rehabilitation before discharge. Elderly persons may require care for an indefinite period, perhaps for the remainder of their lives. These patients, however, no longer need the intensive medical services of the acute-care hospital nor is this facility organized to deal with the "total human configuration." Long-term-care institutions provide the continuum of care required by these patients.

To both minimize public-sector expenditures and to meet the health needs of the patients, chronic care must be viewed as a continuum. What is left undone in one or more sectors of the health-delivery system will have an adverse effect on the other sectors of the total system.[6] Every bed, whether in an acute-care hospital or a long-term-care facility, has an opportunity cost—that is the cost of utilizing that bed is the opportunity sacrificed to treat another patient.

The failure to move a patient from an acute-care-hospital when its services are no longer required denies access and proper treatment to patients' requiring acute hospital care. Similarly, the failure to move patients back into the community, or to lower levels of long-term care when improvement occurs, denies admission to patients who need these levels of care.

When a patient is covered by Medicaid or Medicare, keeping that patient at a higher-than-appropriate level of care is an inefficient use of medical resources and is also costly to the public sector. The higher levels of institutional care are designed "for the purpose of continuing and improving on the stabilization of the patient. The lower levels of care are essentially preventive, to provide people not only with longevity but also with a comfortable life made possible by our concern for them as unique beings."[7]

To efficiently utilize medical resources, and to minimize the public-sector expense that finances a majority of long-term-health care, patients must be placed in facilities appropriate to their needs. Inappropriate placement can interfere with the proper treatment of the patient and deny to other patients access to proper treatment. An integrated, comprehensive network of health-care organizations and services can provide that continuum of care that allows for the efficient utilization of medical resources.

Specialization and Differentiation

The *nursing home,* that all-encompassing term that has been applied to different types of long-term-care facilities, serves a vital function in the continuum of the health-delivery system. However, just as that famous aspirin maker has claimed that "all aspirin is not alike," similarly all nursing homes are not alike. These organizations can be differentiated and classified by the amount and intensity of the medical services their respective patients receive.

To provide that comprehensive continuum of health-care services necessary to meet the health-care needs of the elderly, the types of long-term-care facilities available must be differentiated. Whereas all medical institutions provide services through four major operating divisions, they can be distinguished by the degree to which each institution emphasizes and delivers each of these component services.

The four major operating divisions are (1) the residential-service component including services such as housekeeping, dietary planning, and laundry; (2) the health-services component including all elements of nursing care, medical supervision, medication administration, health screening, and preventive health services; (3) the social component of care including guidance, counseling, activities programming, and spiritual guidance; and (4) the administrative component of care including coordination of the operations of the facility, control of fiscal affairs, and overall management of the organization.[8]

What distinguishes the long-term-care facility from the acute-care hospital is the latter's emphasis on the health-services component in relation to the total services the patient receives. Long-term care facilities can be differentiated among themselves by "the degree to which each of these component divisions is present or absent in proportion to the total service program of the facility and the operational emphasis on that service component."[9] Two major classifications of long-term-health-care organizations are reimbursed by the Medicaid program: (1) the skilled-care institution and (2) the intermediate-care facility.

The Skilled-Care Institution

The skilled-care institution places less emphasis on the health-services component of care than does the acute-care hospital. If a physician determines that a patient will need the constant presence of a skilled nurse, but not necessarily the constant presence of a doctor, the patient should be moved from the acute-care hospital to the skilled-care institution. Since the patient no longer requires the intensive health-service component of care offered by the acute-care hospital, he can be moved to an institution more appropriate to his medical needs and in the process open an acute-care bed to another patient.

Although similarities exist between acute care and extended care, the emphasis placed on the various components of care is different. At the skilled-care institution the social and residential aspects of care become more important in the delivery of services to the patient. The health-services component of care does not receive the intensive emphasis it receives at the acute-care hospital. The health-services component of care is still dominant at the skilled-care institution, but less-frequent physician visits are needed. Instead, the facility concentrates on expert nursing care and rehabilitation services such as accurate control of prescribed medicine, selective therapeutic procedures, and continuous patient observation for physical and mental conditions.

The Intermediate-Care Facility

If the patient's medical condition continues to improve, he may be moved along the continuum of care to the intermediate-care facility. Again, moving the patient to the facility most appropriate to his medical needs makes beds available in the more-intensive health-service facilities and is a more-efficient use of resources.

At the intermediate-care facility the health-service component is at a minimum, and medical needs include supervision, observation, and injections. In these types of residential health organizations, emphasis is placed on preventive medicine designed to maintain patients' health status.

At the intermediate-care facility the residential component, and more importantly, the social component of care should receive primary emphasis. This type of organization is designed to meet the medical needs of the elderly who require more than just residential care yet do not require intensive health services. The intermediate-care facility is designed to meet two objectives in the health-delivery system: (1) to provide the necessary or needed level of health care and (2) to save money by offering a less-expensive alternative to the skilled-care facility.[10]

These objectives can be contradictory. Although the more-ambulatory patient in an intermediate-care facility needs a less-intensive health-services component of care than is required by a counterpart in a skilled-care facility, such care is not necessarily less costly.[11] The social component of care in the ideal intermediate-care facility should include recreational, occupational, and other therapeutic programs designed to give the elderly a sense of purpose and fulfillment. If reimbursement rates for intermediate care are set too low and cover only room, board, and medical expenses, the social component of health care will not be provided. These programs are important to give the elderly institutionalized person a sense of inner dignity so often lost through society's treatment of the institutionalized. These people do no lose their human needs just because they have reached a "golden age." An essential factor in treating the total needs of the elderly institutionalized patient is to recognize the social component of intermediate care and not to view these facilities as simply cost-savings alternatives to skilled care.

Public Spending

In the United States the public sector, primarily through the Medicaid program, has emerged as the dominant third-party purchaser of long-term care. Table 1-1 documents this evolution. During 1971 public funds provided only 38 percent of total revenues used to finance nursing-home care. This percentage increased annually, rising to 55 percent during 1976.

Contrary to what one might expect, the Medicare program, which provides federal health insurance to the elderly, is not the primary purchaser of long-term care. In fact, the program purchases very little care of this type because Medicare regulations permit reimbursement for only 100 days of extended care. The Medicaid program is, however, the most-important third-party purchaser of nursing-home care, providing 50.7 percent of all revenues for this type of care during 1976. Table 1-2 illustrates annual spending levels by both the Medicare and Medicaid programs for long-term care.

Narrowing the analysis of public spending to focus only on the Medicaid program, Medicaid expenditures for nursing-home care have been increasing annually. More importantly, these expenditures have been consuming an increasingly larger percentage of Medicaid funds: rising from 34 percent of all expenditures during 1973 to an estimated 44 percent during 1980, as table 1-3 illustrates. Since 1974 Medicaid expenditures to long-term care facilities have exceeded Medicaid expenditures for general hospital care. Table 1-3 demonstrates the cost significance of long-term care to the Medicaid program, which since 1974 has been the largest Medicaid expenditure category nationally.

Table 1-4 breaks down payments to long-term-care facilities into its skilled- and intermediate-care components, comparing spending on these two items to total Medicaid spending. The table illustrates that an estimated 18 to 26 percent of total Medicaid expenditures went to purchase skilled and intermediate institutional care respectively during 1980. Intermediate-care facilities are consuming an increasingly larger percentage of the Medicaid budget each year. If this trend continues, intermediate-care facilities will shortly consume more Medicaid dollars than acute hospital care, already having surpassed expenditures for skilled care.

Table 1-1
Expenditures for Long-Term Care Facilities
(millions of dollars)

Funds	1971	1972	1973	1974	1975	1976
Source of Funds						
Private	$3,388 (62%)	$3,259 (52%)	$3,386 (51%)	$3,504 (47%)	$4,086 (45%)	$4,744 (45%)
Public	2,058 (38%)	3,015 (48%)	3,264 (49%)	3,946 (53%)	5,014 (55%)	5,856 (55%)
Total	5,466 (100%)	6,274 (100%)	6,650 (100%)	7,450 (100%)	9,100 (100%)	10,600 (100%)
Analysis of Public Funds						
Federal	$1,229 (60%)	$1,745 (58%)	$1,896 (58%)	2,208 (56%)	$2,917 (58%)	$3,417 (58%)
State and Local	829 (40%)	1,271 (42 %)	1,367 (42%)	1,738 (44%)	2,097 (42%)	2,439 (42%)
Total	2,058 (100%)	3,015 (100%)	3,264 (100%)	3,946 (100%)	5,014 (100%)	5,856 (100%)

Source: Data for 1971 and 1972 from U.S., Department of Health, Education, and Welfare, Social Security Administration, *Research and Statistics Note*, 29 November 1974, p. 3. Data for 1973 and 1974 from ibid., 13 May 1975, p. 3. Data for 1975 and 1976 from ibid., 22 December 1976, p. 3.

Note: 1972 initiated Medicaid payments to intermediate-care facilities.

Table 1–2
Public Expenditures for Long-Term Care
(*millions of dollars*)

Year	Medicare	Medicaid
1973	$154	$3,011
1974	224	3,628
1975	285	4,650
1976	326	5,380
1977	362	6,392

Source: Data for 1973 and 1974 from U.S., Department of Health, Education, and Welfare, Social Security Administration, *Compendium of National Health Expenditure Data,* January 1976, pp. 65–66. Data for 1975, 1976, and 1977 from U.S., Department of Health, Education, and Welfare, Social Security Administration, *Social Security Bulletin,* vol. 41, no. 7 (July 1978), pp. 7–9. Medicaid data from U.S., Department of Health, Education, and Welfare, Health Care Finance Administration, Medicaid Bureau, *Data on the Medicaid Program: Eligibility, Services, and Expenditures Fiscal Years 1966–1978,* 1978, p. 31.

Table 1–3
Medicaid Payments to Institutional-Care Facilities
(*millions of dollars*)

Year	Total Medicaid	General Hospital	Long-Term Care
1973	8,810 (100%)	3,113 (35%)	3,011 (34%)
1974	10,149 (100%)	3,399 (33%)	3,628 (36%)
1975	12,245 (100%)	3,915 (32%)	4,650 (38%)
1976	14,245 (100%)	4,518 (32%)	5,380 (38%)
1977	16,300 (100%)	5,128 (31%)	6,392 (39%)
1978	18,134 (100%)	5,581 (31%)	7,583 (42%)
1979 (est.)	20,430 (100%)	6,129 (30%)	8,785 (43%)
1980 (est.)	23,818 (100%)	6,863 (29%)	10,488 (44%)

Source: Data for 1973–1977 from U.S., Department of Health, Education, and Welfare, Health Care Finance Administration, Medicaid Bureau, *Data on the Medicaid Program: Eligibility, Services, and Expenditures Fiscal Years 1966–1978,* 1978, p. 31. Data for 1978, 1979, and 1980 from U.S., Department of Health and Human Services, Health Care Finance Administration, Medicaid Cost Estimates, interview, 23 September 1980.
Note: Long-term care includes payments to both skilled-care and intermediate-care facilities.

Virginia is used to illustrate the rising cost of nursing-home care to state Medicaid programs in table 1–5. The table demonstrates that long-term care has become the major cost item to the Virginia Medicaid program, with 41 percent of program expenditures going to purchase this type of care during 1977.

Table 1-4
Medicaid Payments to Classes of Long-Term-Care Facilities
(*millions of dollars*)

Year	Total Medicaid	Skilled Care	Intermediate Care
1973	$ 8,810 (100%)	$1,849 (21%)	$1,162 (13%)
1974	10,149 (100%)	2,027 (20%)	1,601 (16%)
1975	12,318 (100%)	2,471 (20%)	2,179 (18%)
1976	14,245 (100%)	2,599 (18%)	2,781 (20%)
1977	16,300 (100%)	2,808 (17%)	3,584 (22%)
1978	18,134 (100%)	3,203 (18%)	4,380 (24%)
1979 (est.)	20,430 (100%)	3,677 (18%)	5,108 (25%)
1980 (est.)	23,818 (100%)	4,193 (18%)	6,295 (26%)

Source: Data for 1973-1977 from U.S., Department of Health, Education, and Welfare, Health Care Finance Administration, Medicaid Bureau, *Data on the Medicaid Program: Eligibility, Services, and Expenditures Fiscal Years 1966-1978*, 1978, p. 31. Data for 1978, 1979, and 1980 from U.S., Department of Health and Human Services, Health Care Finance Administration, Medicaid Cost Estimates, interview, 23 September 1980.

Table 1-5
Medicaid Expenditures in Virginia

Year	Total Medicaid Expenditures	Long-Term Care
1972	$ 85,822,990	$ 4,426,469 (5%)
1973	117,220,531	26,275,466 (22%)
1974	141,870,489	43,943,592 (31%)
1975	191,658,300	68,712,814 (36%)
1976	193,518,742	76,255;220 (39%)
1977	248,161,056	102,820,692 (41%)

Source: Data for 1972 from Virginia, Department of Health, *1971 Statistical Annual Report*, 1972, p. 177; for 1973, Virginia, Department of Health, *1972 Statistical Annual Report*, 1973, p. 179; for 1974, Virginia, Department of Health, *1973 Statistical Annual Report*, 1974, p. 198; for 1975, Virginia, Department of Health, *1974 Statistical Annual Report*, 1975, p. 206; for 1976, Virginia, Department of Health, *1975 Statistical Annual Report*, 1976, p. 210; for 1977, Virginia, Department of Health, *1976 Statistical Annual Report*, 1977, p. 208.
Note: During 1972 long-term-care expenditures included only skilled care.

The annual Medicaid expenditure increases by selected spending category are presented in table 1-6. All categories presented in the table have registered increases for the years 1974 through 1980, but spending increases for intermediate care have been phenomenal. If the Medicaid program is to remain financially viable, these expenditure increases must be limited.

Table 1-6
Medicaid Payments for Institutional Inpatient Services
(millions of dollars)

Year	Total Medicaid	Annual Increase	Hospital	Annual Increase	Skilled Care	Annual Increase	Intermediate Care	Annual Increase
1973	$ 8,810	—	$3,113	—	$1,849	—	$1,162	—
1974	10,149	15%	3,399	9%	2,027	9%	1,601	38%
1975	12,318	21	3,915	15	2,471	22	2,179	36
1976	14,245	16	4,518	15	2,599	5	2,781	28
1977	16,300	14	5,128	14	2,808	8	3,584	29
1978	18,134	11	5,581	9	3,203	14	4,380	22
1979 (est.)	20,430	13	6,129	10	3,677	15	5,108	17
1980 (est.)	23,818	17	6,863	12	4,193	14	6,295	23

Source: Data for 1973–1977 from U.S., Department of Health, Education, and Welfare, Health Care Finance Administration, Medicaid Bureau, *Data on the Medicaid Program: Eligibility, Services, and Expenditures Fiscal Years 1966-1978,* 1978, p. 31. Data for 1978, 1979, and 1980 from U.S., Department of Health and Human Services, Health Care Finance Administration, Medicaid Cost Estimates, interview, 23 September 1980.

Issues for Study

Medicaid is a federal grant-in-aid program to state governments, with primary responsibility for the initiation and administration of the Medicaid programs given to the states. These programs are financed through federal/ state cooperation, with the federal contribution at a minimum of 50 percent and a maximum of 83 percent of total program costs in each state. The exact percentage of the federal share depends upon the average per capita income for each state in relation to the per capita income for the entire United States.

Placing the responsibility for Medicaid administration with state governments has resulted in a wide range of reimbursement practices for long-term care. State Medicaid programs adopt payment mechanisms that can differ on at least two dimensions. One dimension concerns the timing for establishing the per diem rate, which can be done either prospectively or retrospectively. If a state program uses prospective-rate determination, then the per diem fee is calculated prior to the time period it is to be applied based on projected costs. Conversely, if a state program uses the retrospective method, then the per diem fee is calculated after the time period to which the rate is applied based on actual costs.

The other dimension to payment mechanisms is concerned with the choice of reimbursement method. The three major categories of payment method used by state Medicaid programs in the past have been the reasonable-cost-related reimbursement, the fixed-rate reimbursement, and the negotiated-rate reimbursement. Within the reasonable-cost-related category many variations exist. Some state programs have called their method *actual cost*. Other states have adopted an actual-cost or reasonable-cost method and then established a maximum ceiling on the per diem fee. One purpose of this study is to describe and compile the Medicaid reimbursement system for skilled care and intermediate care from 1973 through 1977 on a state-by-state basis.

The different reimbursement practices used, coupled with different operating costs in different locations of the United States, have resulted in a wide range of reimbursement rates for long-term care. During 1976 the rates for skilled care ranged from a low of $13.25 per day in Missouri to a high of $60.95 per day in Alaska. In the same year the rates for intermediate care ranged from a low of $11.23 per day in Louisiana to a high of $40.12 per day in Alaska. (See appendix B for a listing of the amount each state paid for the two types of nursing-home care from 1973 through 1977.)

These different reimbursement mechanisms, and the diverse range of per diem rates they produced, generated tremendous debate over payment-related issues both within the health-care community and the government. What effects have Medicaid reimbursement practices had on the cost and utilization of long-term care? Are these different reimbursement methods associated with different levels of cost? Do the different payment methods affect the access by Medicaid patients to nursing-home care in the United States?

To assess the impact of reimbursement on cost, the various states are grouped according to reimbursement methods. Average per diem costs for each type of care are calculated for each reimbursement mechanism for the years 1973 through 1977. Average annual cost changes are also calculated for each reimbursement method. Through statistical analysis we determine whether the average per diem cost, and the annual cost changes, differ significantly among the different reimbursement methods.

Utilization indexes are also developed to measure the use of long-term care by Medicaid patients. Again the states are grouped according to reimbursement methods for each year from 1973 through 1976. Through the use of statistical analysis we determine whether the access to nursing-home care by Medicaid patients differs among reimbursement methods.

The nursing-home industry claims it cannot deliver adequate care because of inadequate Medicaid payments. Critics of the long-term-care industry, which is comprised mostly of profit-seeking businesses, claim that nursing homes are reaping excessive profits. The Senate Finance Committee has been concerned that the diverse Medicaid reimbursement system might have resulted in some state programs' paying too much for long-term care and other state programs' paying too little to insure the delivery of adequate quality care.

This controversy led to federal legislation that attempted to standardize the reimbursement mechanism for nursing-home care. The debate focused on that dimension of payment dealing with reimbursement methods. In 1972, PL 92–603 (Section 249) amended the Social Security Act to require that all state Medicaid programs reimburse long-term care facilities on a reasonable-cost-related basis, effective 1 July 1976. What prompted the creation of this law requiring reasonable-cost-related reimbursement? Which political actors, both formal and informal, were involved in the development? What legal and political controversies did Section 249 generate? The development of PL 92–603 (Section 249) in the public-policy process is traced in chapter 5.

The effects of prospective- and retrospective-rate determination on the cost and utilization of nursing-home care are analyzed. The two methods for setting rates are defined, and the pros and cons of each technique are described. Thus the major objective of this rate-setting research is to assess empirically the merits of each set of arguments and to make recommendations. Can the prospective-rate-setting device reduce Medicaid expenditures without adversely affecting the access of Medicaid patients to long-term care?

The major focus of this study is to describe and analyze the Medicaid payment system for nursing-home care to discover reimbursement practices that can increase both the quality of care and the efficiency of its delivery. As the number of elderly Americans increases in the future, and as long-term-care costs continue to rise, Medicaid expenditures for nursing-home care will skyrocket. Can reimbursement practices be developed to help contain these soaring costs? Will the profit motive help or hinder this effort? Can the profit motive be harnessed to increase both the quality of care and the efficiency of its delivery? These are all questions this study analyzes and attempts to answer.

Notes

1. Arthur Isack, "Federal Government Involvement in Training Medical Directors of Long-Term-Care Facilities," *Journal of the American Geriatrics Society* 21:261.

2. Ethel Shanas, "Factors Affecting the Care of the Patient," *Journal of the American Geriatrics Society* 21:395.

3. U.S., Department of Health, Education, and Welfare, Social Security Administration, *Research and Statistics Note* DHEW Publication, no. SSA 75–11701 (13 May 1975), p. 3.

4. Neil Gaynes, "A Logic to Long-Term Care," *Gerontologist* 13(Autumn 1973):278.

5. Samuel Levey et al., "An Appraisal of Nursing Home Care," *Journal of Gerontology* 28:223.

6. Richard Nauen, "A Method for Planning for the Care of Long-Term Patients," *American Journal of Public Health* 58(November 1968):2119.

7. Irving Schor, M.D., "Fitting Long-Term Care to the Patient's Need," *Geriatrics* 29(February 1974):164.

8. Gaynes, "A Logic to Long-Term Care," pp. 277–78.

9. Ibid., p. 278.

10. Kenneth Frank, "Government Support of Nursing Home Care," *New England Journal of Medicine* 257:541.

11. Ibid., p. 541.

2

The Nursing-Home Industry: Profit, Medicaid, and Reimbursement

The skilled care and the intermediate care described in chapter 1 are delivered by a large and growing long-term-care industry. The growth rate of the industry has been impressive. Total expenditures on nursing-home care in the United States were $28 million in 1940, $178 million in 1950, and $480 million in 1960. With the initiation of the Medicare and Medicaid programs in the mid-1960s, long-term-care expenditures jumped from $1.3 billion in 1965 to $3.8 billion in 1970.[1] A *Business Week* study estimated total long-term-care revenues at $14.5 billion for 1978.[2] These revenue figures illustrate that the nursing-home industry is one of America's largest and fastest-growing businesses.

In addition to increasing revenues, other factors indicate the growth of this industry. For example, between 1960 and 1970 the number of long-term-care facilities increased from 9,582 to 23,000; the number of beds increased from 331,000 to 1,099,000; and the number of patients increased from 290,000 to 900,000.[3] As discussed in chapter 1, government programs, particularly Medicaid, have provided much of the revenues to fuel this phenomenal growth.

Profit versus Nonprofit Institutions

Institutional long-term care is delivered by either nonprofit or profit (proprietary) organizations. Nonprofit institutions can be either privately owned, such as religious or fraternal homes, or government owned. Nationwide, approximately 73 percent of the long-term-care institutions are operated on a profit basis, and nearly 75 percent of the more than one million institutionalized long-term-care patients are in proprietary facilities.[4] Considerable controversy and debate has been generated over the desirability of the predominantly for-profit orientation of the long-term-care industry. Can profit-seeking health-care institutions deliver quality care at a reasonable cost? Or will patient care be sacrificed to the pursuit of profits? Compounding the fear of the profit motive in the delivery of nursing-home care is the increasing importance of the large, long-term-health-care corporation. Some health-care experts fear that the corporate structure and the profit motive may adversely affect the quality of the care delivered.

One Canadian health-care official has stated his concern for the growing financial motivation in the delivery of long-term care. "It seems to be an unfortunate sign of the times that more people are becoming more interested in the financial return than in the service they are providing. . . . The quality of care may well deteriorate and become less personal under these circumstances."[5]

Some health-care investigators have charged that this growing financial motivation has led to profiteering at the expense of the quality of care the institutionalized elderly receive. One study concludes that the nursing-home industry delivers poor patient care and receives excessively high profits. The author of this study further states: "One conclusion is inescapable: nursing homes are a very lucrative business. Despite the pleas of poverty from operators caught cutting corners in the care of their patients, despite the many variations I have heard on the theme of Saul Tobias [a nursing-home operator] and his vending machine—give us a dime and we'll give you a dime's worth of service—it became abundantly clear to me that nursing-home operators are getting rich at the expense of their patients and the taxpayers."[6]

A report to the AFL-CIO Executive Council on the conditions in American long-term-care facilities states:

> FACT: Public funding accounts for about $1 out of every $2 in nursing-home expenditures, with most of that money coming from the Medicaid program and going to private, profit-making nursing homes.

> FACT: In recent years there have been scores of investigations, indictments, and convictions for fraud against Medicaid, most of which have been committed by private, for-profit nursing homes.

> FACT: Most of the abuses in terms of patient care uncovered by the AFL-CIO investigation and by several other inquiries came from private, profit-making nursing homes.

> One common thread unites these three facts and leads to an inescapable conclusion: most of the problems in nursing homes can be traced to the profit motive, which is incompatible with social programs. Ultimately, in order to correct the problems of nursing homes, profit must be eliminated from the nursing-home industry. . . .

> RECOMMENDATIONS: Gradual phasing out of private, for-profit, nursing homes and replacement by nonprofit, religious, or government ownership.[7]

The Subcommittee on Long-Term Care of the Senate Special Committee on Aging issued a report in 1974 revealing important nursing-home abuses. Among these abuses were "negligence leading to death and injury," "unsanitary conditions," "poor food," and "reprisals against those who complained."[8] The same report, which discussed the nursing-home industry in general (not just proprietary institutions), estimated that the number of substandard facilities ranged from 30–80 percent, with substandard defined as "a violation of one or more standards which creates a life-threatening situation."

Many critics of proprietary long-term-care facilities have charged that the profit motive is responsible for this condition and has caused profiteering, abuse, Medicaid fraud, and the delivery of low-quality health care.

Are proprietary institutions really making excessive profits and delivering low-quality care? Since public revenues finance over 50 percent of the institutional long-term care in the United States, are the taxpayers purchasing inferior-quality care and contributing to excess profits when their public revenues purchase long-term care from proprietary institutions? If evidence supports these indictments against the proprietary providers of long-term care, then government should take steps to eliminate the profit motive from the industry as the AFL-CIO recommends.

Profits and Nursing Homes

How profitable are the long-term-care corporations in the United States, and how do these profitability levels compare to other U.S. industries? One indicator that large nursing-home chains are not making large profits comes from an article in *Business Week* that states that these companies are having problems securing financial backing from lenders.[9] Table 2–1 summarizes the profitability of selected U.S. industries and compares their profit margins to the profit margins for a long-term-care index developed for this analysis. Profit margin is an expression of after-tax profits as a percentage of total sales.

The long-term corporate index was developed based on a discussion in *Modern Health Care* of the largest nursing-home chains in the United States.[10] Not all the companies listed in the article were included in the index because some, such as ARA Services, Inc., are large multidivision companies. Long-term-care services are only one component of the operations of these companies, and it was not possible to isolate long-term-care sales and profit data. (See appendix A for an annual summary of the profitability of the corporations included in the long-term-care index.)

The industries presented in table 2–1 were selected for purposes of comparison from the annual review of U.S. industry by *Business Week*.[11] The industries selected for presentation are only a fraction of all the industries presented by this business journal. However, the industry composite presented in the table summarizes the profitability of approximately 1,200 companies from all the industries surveyed by *Business Week* in its annual review of U.S. corporate performance.

Table 2–1
Profitability of Selected U.S. Industries: After-Tax Profit Margins

Industry	1979	1978	1977	1976	1975	1974	1973
Long-term-care index	2.6%	2.9%	3.2%	1.0%	1.4%	0.4%	0.9%
1,200 composite of industries	5.5	5.4	5.2	5.3	4.8	5.3	5.9
Airlines	1.7	5.0	3.7	2.1	(loss)	2.5	1.9
Appliances	2.2	3.8	4.6	4.1	1.9	1.8	4.5
Automotive	2.8	4.0	4.5	4.4	1.9	2.2	4.7
Chemical	6.4	6.0	5.8	6.6	6.6	7.7	7.5
Drugs	9.7	9.8	9.5	9.0	9.1	9.3	9.8
Electronics	5.7	5.7	5.4	5.1	10.8	4.0	4.6
Food processing	3.1	3.1	3.2	3.3	3.1	3.1	3.0
Leisure time	8.6	8.5	5.6	5.6	5.3	3.7	3.7
Office equipment/computers	9.6	10.3	10.1	9.9	9.5	9.5	10.0
Tobacco	6.0	5.6	5.4	5.2	5.5	6.5	6.3
Trucking	3.3	4.3	4.4	4.7	3.9	3.8	3.9
Utilities	9.7	10.6	10.8	10.9	10.6	11.1	12.3

Source: Data for 1979 from *Business Week*, 17 March 1980, pp. 81–116; for 1978, *Business Week*, 19 March 1979, pp. 69–104; for 1977, *Business Week*, 20 March 1978, pp. 79–114; for 1976, *Business Week*, 21 March 1977, pp. 77–112; for 1975, *Business Week*, 22 March 1976, pp. 6–104; for 1974, *Business Week*, 24 March 1975, pp. 57–91; for 1973, *Business Week*, 9 March, 1974, pp. 80–108.

Note: The information for the long-term-care index was gathered from corporate 10–K reports. See appendix A.

Table 2-1 clearly demonstrates that the nursing-home chains analyzed, which were among the largest in the United States, are not making excessive profits as their critics have charged. This conclusion becomes even more pronounced when the long-term-care index is compared to the general industry composite. The composite profit margin for the 1,200 largest U.S. companies always far exceeded the profit margins of the long-term-care chains analyzed from 1973-1979.

The profit margins of utilities, which were consistently 10 percent and over, far exceeded the profit margins of the nursing-home chains, whose highest margin was 3.2 percent in 1977. In the health-care area, drug companies consistently achieved margins of over 9 percent. In a private-enterprise system high profit margins are the necessary incentives to attract new capital into an industry to expand its output. These relatively low profit margins for nursing-home corporations may explain why shortages of long-term-care beds exist in many areas of the United States today. The profitability analysis of nursing-home corporations presented in table 2-1 clearly demonstrates that these companies generate lower rates of profit for their owners than the average U.S. corporation.

Cost of Care and Type of Ownership

Related to the concept of profitability is the charge that proprietary long-term-care facilities seek their profits by charging relatively higher prices. If for-profit nursing homes charge a significantly higher price than nonprofit facilities, and the quality of care between the two types of ownership is similar, then perhaps the Medicaid program should purchase long-term care from nonprofit homes to minimize program costs or to attempt to remove the profit motive from the nursing-home industry.

A study published in the *American Journal of Public Health* concluded that in Massachusetts a significant relationship did exist between the type of ownership and the cost of care. The study concluded that proprietary ownership was "generally associated with lower costs in contrast to high costs in nonprofit homes."[12]

A 1968 study of Minnesota long-term-care facilities revealed that the type of ownership had no significant effect on the cost of care.[13]

Another study of Massachusetts facilities for both 1965 and 1969 revealed no statistically significant difference in the cost of long-term care for the three types of ownership studied.[14] Table 2-2 summarizes these findings. An interesting fact to note from the table is not only the greater per diem cost of long-term care delivered by the nonprofit organization but also the higher rate of cost increase for nonprofit care between 1965 and 1969.

Finally, a study of proprietary and nonproprietary long-term-care facilities in Virginia concluded that proprietary institutions delivered care less expensively, although the difference was not statistically significant.[15] Table 2-3 presents the results of this analysis.

Based on the studies surveyed, either no statistically significant difference exists in the prices charged by profit and nonprofit nursing homes, or if a significant difference exists, then the proprietary facilities are less expensive. Even the AFL-CIO study, which is critical of proprietary long-term-care institutions, admits that profit-making nursing homes have an average per diem cost that is less than nonprofit homes.

The evidence suggests that proprietary long-term-care facilities neither charge excessive prices nor do they make excessive profits. However, at least one more variable must be explored before the proprietary long-term-care industry can be given a clean bill of health relative to the nonprofit segment of the industry. Is there a difference between the quality of care delivered by proprietary and nonproprietary long-term-care institutions?

Quality of Care and Type of Ownership

A Canadian health-care official was quoted earlier in this chapter as stating that "the quality of care may well deteriorate" when nursing-home care is delivered by profit-making institutions. Since on average the profit institutions charge a lower per diem price than do nonprofit institutions, do the owners and administrators make their profits by delivering lower-quality care? Does a correlation exist between the different types of ownership and the quality of care? Various studies have been undertaken to determine whether a statistically significant variance exists in the quality of care by the type of ownership.

In the case of long-term care, it is difficult to measure or quantify the quality of care received by a patient. The studies cited in this section have all used proxy measures to evaluate the quality of the care delivered. Proxy measures are analytical tools used to generate information about a condition or situation. If certain health-care services are given to a patient, then this may indicate that higher-quality care is received than if these services are not given.

The value of a proxy measure depends upon the proved linkage or correlation between the proxy measure and the delivery of high-quality care. The studies reviewed here have not established this linkage. Therefore, these studies really analyze the type of ownership in relation to the range of services delivered rather than the quality of care delivered. However, the studies are useful to determine whether the profit motive has encouraged proprietary institutions to reduce the quantity of services delivered in order to minimize costs and increase profits.

Table 2–2
Cost of Care by Type of Ownership for Long-Term-Care Facilities in Massachusetts

Year	Average Per Diem Total Cost of Care		
	Noncorporate Proprietary	Corporate Proprietary	Corporate Nonproprietary
1965	$ 8.34	$ 9.14	$11.07
1969	11.91 (43%)	14.97 (64%)	20.13 (82%)

Source: Samuel Levey et al., "An Appraisal of Nursing-Home Care," *Journal of Gerontology* 28(February 1973):222–28.
Note: The percentage increases of 1969 over the 1965 rates follow the 1969 rates in parenthesis.

Table 2–3
Cost of Care by Type of Ownership in Virginia, 1974

Facility	Average Per Diem Cost
Intermediate care	
Proprietary	$18.69
Nonproprietary	19.97
Skilled care	
Proprietary	29.93
Nonproprietary	32.19

Source: Robert J. Buchanan, "Public Policy and Long-Term Care," (Master's thesis, University of Virginia, 1976), p. 41.

A 1973 study that analyzed the quality of care in Massachusetts was published in the *Journal of Gerontology* and concluded that no statistically significant difference existed in the services delivered between types of ownership.[17] The study identified what the researchers considered to be the nine major components of care. When these major components of care were analyzed by type of ownership, no significant difference was evident between the services delivered and the type of ownership. The authors of this Massachusetts study reached a conclusion that is significant to Medicaid officials. The researchers noticed a "marked increase in the levels of the services" delivered by nursing homes between 1965 and 1969. They attributed these improvements in the delivery of care to modifications in rate-setting and enforcement programs in Massachusetts. This information suggests that the Medicaid program, in its dual role as health-care purchaser and as regulator/licensor of health-care facilities, can influence what services long-term-care institutions deliver to patients.

A 1969 study conducted by Anderson and Stone demonstrated that the type of ownership had "little effect" on the comprehensiveness of staff and personnel services, facilities, or patient activity delivered by long-term-care institutions. The authors concluded "that the profit motive does not necessarily affect the likelihood of the presence of quality-of-care indicators."[18]

Another study by Anderson and Holmberg in Minnesota in 1968 focused on the differences in services delivered by proprietary and nonproprietary facilities.[19] The three areas studied were facilities, staff and personnel, and programs.

Facilities

A comparison of physical facilities by type of ownership revealed the most differences, with nonproprietary institutions having more beds, more buildings, and more floors in the buildings. A study by Penchansky and Taubenhaus stated that an institution with a small number of beds has an adverse effect on the quality of care because the small nursing home cannot enjoy economies of scale. The low number of patients and the correspondingly low revenue of the facility limit the specialized personnel, staff, and therapy services the institution can afford to deliver because per-patient costs of these services are too high.[20] However, proprietary institutions in Minnesota averaged 51.41 beds per institution (72.76 beds for nonproprietary), which is higher than the 15–30–bed size mentioned by Penchansky and Taubenhaus as adversely affecting quality.

Staff and Personnel

Due to the fact that nursing and medical services can affect the health levels of patients, differences in staffing by type of ownership could indicate quality differences. The study revealed no statistically significant variance by type of ownership in the number of employees; in the number of hours worked per week; or in the positions of registered nurses, nurses aides, dieticians, occupational therapists, or physical therapists. Nonproprietary facilities had a physician on call a significantly greater number of hours per week than did proprietary institutions. With this exception, however, no statistically significant difference was evident in the health-care services delivered by type of ownership.

Programs

Nursing homes customarily provide various programs to improve the patients' "psychological maintenance" and rehabilitation. Type of ownership had no significant effect on birthday celebrations, communal dining, entertainment programs, hobby workshops, and other programs. The effects of ownership were significant, however, in two areas: (1) proprietary homes had a greater percentage of patients participating in holiday celebrations, and (2) nonproprietary homes had more residents making purchases at the stores the institutions provide.

In summary, based on the studies reviewed, no significant difference appears between the services that proprietary and nonproprietary nursing homes deliver. If the services delivered can be used as reliable proxy measures for the quality of care, which these researchers assume but have not proved, then there is no difference in the quality of care delivered by type of ownership.

Critics have charged that proprietary long-term-care facilities, driven by the profit motive, deliver costly, lower-quality care while making excessive profits. The studies reviewed refute the charges that the quality of care in profit-making nursing homes is lower in quality than that delivered by nonprofit facilities. Per diem costs in proprietary institutions tend to be lower when they differ from the per diem costs of nonproprietary nursing homes. Profitability measures such as profit as a percentage of sales for proprietary long-term-care chains are lower than for U.S. industry in general. Transforming the long-term-care industry into a nonprofit industry would not necessarily increase the quality of care, but it may in fact increase the cost of care.

The Market System and Long-Term Care

In some respects the market system and the profit motive have worked well in the delivery of institutional long-term care. The profit motive has provided incentives to proprietary facilities to deliver long-term care more efficiently to increase profits. The market system, competition, and profits have also provided somewhat of an incentive for long-term-care facilities to provide high-quality care to attract patients. Jack Davis, President of National Health Enterprises, states that "quality care is our best marketing tool."[21]

Although the profit motive and competition may encourage proprietary long-term-care facilities to minimize costs to increase profits, the market mechanism breaks down as the sole protector of the quality of care. One reason for this breakdown is that in the majority of cases, the "consumer" of long-term care (the patient) is different from the "purchaser" of these services (Medicaid).

In most economic transactions these dual roles of consumer and purchaser are linked in the same person. If the consumer is satisfied with past purchases, then the consumer will continue to purchase the good or service in the future. Previous satisfaction encourages future purchases. In a market system firms react to consumer preferences and deliver the type and quality of goods or services that receive sufficient dollar votes from consumers to generate a profit. Here Adam Smith's invisible-hand theory is at work—that is, all economic actors, pursuing their self-interest, act in a way that maximizes the benefit of all.

In the case of a market approach to long-term care, this invisible hand has become somewhat arthritic in its ability to guarantee the quality of care. As mentioned earlier, one Senate study has estimated that 30–80 percent of all nursing homes are substandard. Studies have documented that the quality of care does not vary with the type of ownership. Proprietary and nonproprietary nursing homes alike can be substandard. With the separation of consumer from purchaser, the ability of the consumer to influence and regulate the quality of care is reduced. The nursing-home patients themselves compound this problem. As a group they tend to be old (average age 82, ill (average 3.8 disabilities per person), and mentally deficient to some extent (estimates indicate that 55–80 percent of institutional long-term-care patients are mentally impaired).[22] At best, nursing-home residents have difficulty in making rational choices about the complex medical care they require or in evaluating its quality. At worst they are prey for the wolves of the industry.

The residents of long-term-care facilities cannot exercise consumer sovereignty, which states that consumers know their best interests and will act accordingly. For this reason the market cannot be left alone to guarantee that the residents of long-term-care institutions, whether for profit or nonprofit, receive high-quality care. The Medicaid program, as the major purchaser of nursing-home care in the United States, has a major responsibility to the taxpayer who finances this care and to the patients who consume this care to guarantee the delivery of high-quality health care.

This study advocates a role for private enterprise in the delivery of long-term-health care but does not deny that individual nursing-home operators and administrators have "ripped off" elderly patients and the Medicaid program. The Bergman scandals in New York State, probably the most notorious of the many nursing-home scandals, should remind everyone concerned with long-term care that greed can cause humans to inhumanely exploit fellow humans. The Bergmans of the nursing-home industry illustrate the need for more-effective public-sector monitoring of the delivery of institutional long-term care.

The challenge that faces the Medicaid program and its administrators is to find methods to harness the profit motive to promote efficiency while protecting against patient abuse and the delivery of low-quality care. Regulation and reimbursement are at least two approaches toward this challenge, with reimbursement offering the greatest promise.

Notes

1. Kenneth Frauendorf, "Competition and Public Policy in the Nursing Home Industry," *Journal of Economic Issues* 11(September 1977):608.

2. "Nursing the Nursing Homes Back to Health," *Business Week,* 5 December 1977, p. 66.

3. U.S., Congress, Senate, Subcommittee on Long-Term Care *Nursing Home Care in the United States—Failure in Public Policy,* 93rd Cong. 2d. session, 1974, p. 21.

4. A Report to the AFL-CIO Executive Council, *America's Nursing Homes, Profit in Misery,* 21 February 1977, p. 4.

5. Will Roven, "The Changing Environment of the 70s," *Canadian Hospital* 49(January 1972):49.

6. Mary Mendelson, *Tender Loving Greed* (New York: Alfred A. Knopf, 1974), p. 29.

7. AFL-CIO, *America's Nursing Homes,* pp. 18–19. Reprinted with permission.

8. U.S., Congress, Senate, Special Committee on Aging, Subcommittee on Long-Term Care, *Nursing Home Care,* p. 21.

9. *Business Week,* "Nursing the Nursing Homes," p. 66.

10. Maria Traska, "Proprietary Chains Operated 20% More Beds During 1977," *Modern Health Care* 8(June 1978):38, 42–43.

11. *Business Week,* 20 March 1978, pp. 79–114.

12. "Nursing Homes in Transition," *American Journal of Public Health* 65:68–70.

13. Nancy Anderson and R.H. Holmberg, "Implications of Ownership for Long-Term Care," *Medical Care* 6(July–August 1968):300–07.

14. Samuel Levey et al., "An Appraisal of Nursing Home Care," *Journal of Gerontology* 28(February 1973):222–28.

15. Robert Buchanan, "Public Policy and Long-Term Care" (Master's thesis, University of Virginia, 1976), p. 41.

16. AFL-CIO, *America's Nursing Homes,* p. 4.

17. Samuel Levey et al., "An Appraisal of Nursing Home Care."

18. Nancy Anderson and Lana Stone, "Nursing Homes: Research and Public Policy," *Gerontologist* 9(Autumn 1969):217.

19. Nancy Anderson and R.H. Holmberg, "Implications of Ownership."

20. Roy Penchansky and Leon Taubenhaus, "Institutional Factors Affecting the Quality of Care in Nursing Homes," *Geriatrics* (July 1965):595–97.

21. *Business Week,* "Nursing the Nursing Homes," p. 70.

22. U.S., Congress, Senate, Subcommittee on Long-Term Care, *Nursing Home Care,* p. 15.

3

Medicaid Reimbursement Methods

The Medicaid Program

In 1965 the Social Security Act was amended to include Title XVIII and Title XIX, creating the Medicare and Medicaid programs, respectively. The Medicare program is designed to assist the elderly in obtaining health-care services. Medicaid is a federal grant-in-aid program to the state governments to provide health care to low-income people.

Medicaid has been called the "sleeper" of the 1965 Social Security legislation.[1] Congressional debate over the Social Security amendments had focused almost entirely on the Medicare program. The Medicaid program was created without much debate in the federal policy process. The Medicaid "architects never delineated clear goals" for the program.[2] Also, Medicaid policymakers had "no clear sense of the potential costs of the program or of the impact of pumping vast sums of federal money into the private sector of the medical market."[3]

Title XIX requires that the states have the primary responsibility for the initiation and administration of their Medicaid programs. These programs are financed through federal/state cooperation, with the federal contribution at a minimum of 50 percent and a maximum of 83 percent of the total program cost in each state.[4] The exact percentage of federal financial participation in each state program is based upon the average per capita income of each state in relation to the per capita income of the entire United States for the three most-recent calendar years.[5]

Federal requirements for state participation in the Medicaid program mandate that state programs must provide coverage of inpatient and outpatient hospitalization and laboratory, x-ray, physician, home-health, and skilled-care services.[6] PL 92-223, effective in 1972, amended the Social Security Act to permit states the option to reimburse intermediate-care facilities under their Medicaid program.[7] The amount to be reimbursed and the duration of coverage for these basic services are left to the discretion of each state program.

Medicaid's Impact

The Medicaid program has had a major impact on the U.S. health-care system for over a decade. The program has dramatically improved the ability of the poor to act as consumers of medical services. According to the Department of Health and Human Services (DHHS; formerly the Department of Health, Education, and Welfare) in 1964, prior to the Medicaid program approximately 25 percent of the nation's poor had not been examined by a physician in the previous two years. By 1974 the percentage of the nation's poor who had not seen a doctor in the previous two years had fallen to 17 percent.[8] About 20 percent of the U.S. population has received some type of medical care through the Medicaid program. Finally, due to the impact of the Medicaid program, the commissioner of Program Planning and Evaluation at the DHHS has concluded that "the poor are using health services at about the same rate as the nonpoor."[9] In effect, the Medicaid program has removed poverty as a barrier to obtaining health-care services.

The Medicaid program has removed the lack of purchasing power as an obstacle to obtaining health care but at a substantial cost to the public sector. For 1980, the Medicaid program had estimated expenditures of $23.8 billion, up from $14.2 billion in 1976 and $8.8 billion in 1973.[10] (See table 1-3 for total annual Medicaid program costs.)

The cost increases for federal health-care programs have been so great that one DHHS official was quoted as saying: "The health-cost increases will put a squeeze on every other program budget in town."[11]

The increasing cost of the Medicaid program also drains the financial resources of the states, as they must directly finance part of their respective state Medicaid programs. These upward-cost pressures have forced more than twenty states to decrease reimbursement levels, cut back on benefits, and/or tighten eligibility requirements in an effort to balance their budgets.[12]

One of the major, and fastest-growing, expenditure categories in the Medicaid program is reimbursement to long-term-care facilities. During 1980, estimates indicate that 44 percent of Medicaid's total annual expenditures went to purchase institutional long-term care—up from 34 percent in 1973. (See table 1-3 for long-term care's percentage of total annual Medicaid expenditures. See table 1-6 for annual Medicaid-expenditure increases for institutional care.) These upward-cost pressures have forced various states to attempt to restrict their Medicaid-program expenditures for nursing-home care. Examples of these cost-reduction attempts in the long-term area of Medicaid are: Nevada has dropped intermediate-care coverage for tuberculosis; Alabama, Georgia, and Wisconsin have reduced the "personal-needs allowance" of Medicaid patients in long-term-care facilities; Georgia has also decreased Medicaid payments to nursing homes so they do not exceed payments for the same type of care by the Medicare program; and Alabama has placed an upper limit on reimbursement rates to skilled-care and intermediate-care facilities.[13]

One opportunity to limit Medicaid program costs is to limit Medicaid expenditures for long-term care. Through reimbursement practices the Medicaid program has not only the opportunity to control long-term-care costs but also to promote efficiency and influence the quality of care. The subject of Medicaid long-term-care reimbursement has generated much controversy between the federal and state governments and between government and the long-term-care industry.

Medicaid Reimbursement and Long-Term Care

Medicaid reimbursement policies for long-term care have an important influence on the public-spending levels for the Medicaid program. In addition, since the state Medicaid programs have become the predominant purchasers of nursing-home care, Medicaid reimbursement policies also influence prices paid by private purchasers, efficiency in production, quality of care, and the comprehensiveness of the range of services available to Medicaid recipients.[14] Due to this major impact of payment methods on long-term care, Medicaid reimbursement has become an important public-policy issue.

Goals for Reimbursement Methods

Before discussing the merits of actual reimbursement methods or proposing reimbursement reforms, we must identify the goals of a reimbursement system to be used as a framework for analysis. A study by Ruchlin, Levey, and Muller states that a "viable and acceptable reimbursement plan should seek to accomplish and/or facilitate four major goals."[15] These goals are:

1. To develop a reimbursement system which recognizes and adequately compensates for the fact that the health status of patients consists of physical, psychological, and social components, which determine patient needs in the long-term-care setting. Emphasis should be placed on arriving at a measure of the effectiveness of care in relation to patient needs and patient mix, rather than on the range of services provided patients at any given facility.

Basically, this first goal states that reimbursement levels should be associated with the effectiveness of care in meeting the patient's health needs rather than with basing remuneration solely on the quantity of services delivered. Was the care delivered necessary and effective in terms of the patient's health status? This is a more-important question in terms of promoting economic efficiency and increasing the quality of care than if remuneration was simply based on how much care was delivered.

2.   To facilitate the development of a comprehensive range of health-care services and facilities, including alternatives to institutionalization, to assure that patients are receiving the correct care.

The implementation of this goal would require many state programs to expand the range of long-term-care services that are reimbursable under the Medicaid programs. An example is the delivery of geriatrics day care. Some nursing-home residents do not require institutional care, yet because less-intensive long-term-care services are not Medicaid reimbursable, and the patient cannot afford to purchase the alternative care directly, residence in an intermediate-care facility usually results in Medicaid's absorbing the increased cost of care. If day care was universally Medicaid reimbursable, the patient could utilize that service. A comprehensive range of Medicaid-reimbursable services would facilitate proper patient placement in the long-term-health-care continuum and also utilize Medicaid revenues more efficiently.

3.   To apply continuous pressure for improving operating efficiency.
4.   To develop a system where the providers of care perceive cost containment and efficiency in production as being in the best interests of their institution.

Another health-care analyst has identified the following goals as "appropriate for a reimbursement system":

1.   Encouragement of efficient provision of services.
2.   Avoidance of inducements to admit patients who can be served more economically through home-care services.
3.   Encouragement of the maintenance of publicly determined quality standards.
4.   Provision of a competitive rate of return on capital investment in an efficiently run institution.[16]

These two sets of reimbursement objectives can be synthesized since they are closely related:

1.   The reimbursement method should encourage the efficient delivery of institutional long-term care by creating incentives in the reimbursement method to minimize the costs of delivering care.

2. The reimbursement method should encourage the delivery only of those services necessary to increase or maintain the patient's health status. To promote the delivery of quality care, the reimbursement method ideally should include a measure of the effectiveness of care, and payment levels should be related to that quality measure.

3. The reimbursement method should encourage the delivery of long-term care that is consistent in quality with Medicaid-determined standards. A quality-of-care measure, as discussed in the previous goal, would aid in this endeavor.

4. To further encourage the efficient utilization of Medicaid resources and to provide for the delivery of proper care, the state Medicaid programs should reimburse a comprehensive range of long-term-health-care services including alternatives to institutional care.

5. Proprietary long-term-care institutions should be allowed to make a competitive rate of return on investment.

With reference to goal 2, an attempt to include an effectiveness-of-care measure in the reimbursement method is probably the most-utopian objective of reimbursement reform. Ideally, payment for each long-term-care patient should be linked to an individual-patient effectiveness-of-care measure. Linking reimbursement levels for individual patient care to the effectiveness of the care received would provide strong incentives to the nursing home to deliver quality care efficiently. The incentive to deliver quality care is obvious because if the patient effectiveness-of-care measure does not reflect the desired results in the patient's health status, then reimbursement would be reduced. Also, to minimize costs the nursing home has the incentive to deliver only those health-care services that will positively affect the patient's health status.

A potential for problems exists with measuring the effectiveness of care the long-term-care patients receive. What criteria are to be used in determining if the care delivered is effective in achieving desirable patient-health outcomes? Would the administrative costs of evaluating the effectiveness of care for each patient be prohibitive?

The administrative and methodological costs of linking payment for individual patients to effectiveness-of-care measures are probably prohibitively high. A more-practical solution may be to develop quality-of-care measures, by different classifications of care, for each institution participating in the Medicaid program. This quality-of-care index would measure how closely the institution fulfilled Medicaid's quality and safety standards. Medical research should be conducted to identify which long-term-health-care services have a positive effect on long-term-care patients. Then the Medicaid program could require that these services be delivered by nursing homes to qualify for Medicaid certification. A quality-of-care index could then be used to link patient reimbursement with each facility's quality-performance measure.

Goal 5 states that long-term-care institutions should be allowed the opportunity to make a competitive rate of return on investment. However, this does not mean that nursing homes should be guaranteed an X-percentage return on investment or sales as their profit. To guarantee firms a certain percentage of profits would weaken efficiency incentives to minimize costs in the quest for profits. However, the reimbursement method should not penalize efficient long-term-care facilities by placing profit limits on what they can earn. With strict quality control through Medicaid inspection and certification to guarantee quality of care, nursing homes should not be discouraged from being efficient—maintaining quality while minimizing the costs of production. The Medicaid reimbursement method should reward efficiency by allowing increased profits.

Medicaid Reimbursement Methods

These five reimbursement goals provide a framework to analyze past reimbursement methods used by the various state Medicaid programs. Prior to the passage of PL 92–603 (Section 249), which requires that all state Medicaid programs reimburse long-term-care facilities on a "reasonable-cost-related basis," the states were free to use any reimbursement method for long-term care. This resulted in a wide range of reimbursement rates and a number of reimbursement methods for nursing-home care (see appendix B).

Although there were variations on each major approach, the reimbursement methods used by the state Medicaid programs prior to PL 92–603 (Section 249) fell into three major categories: (1) the reasonable-cost-related method, (2) the fixed-rate method, and (3) the negotiated-rate method.

Reasonable-Cost-Related Method. Various state Medicaid programs used many different versions of the reasonable-cost-related method. Some states used the Medicare program's (Title XVIII) definition of reasonable cost. Other states used their own definition of reasonable cost and placed a limit on their payments so as not to exceed Medicare payments for similar services. A few states call their reimbursement method *actual cost* or *cost-plus-profit factor*. In all cases the principle is the same: to relate reimbursement to the costs incurred by the nursing home in the delivery of care.

Statistical analysis revealed no significant difference for cost and utilization variables among these reasonable-cost-related variations, giving empirical support to grouping these variations together. (See appendix J for the results of the statistical analysis performed on the reasonable-cost-related variations.)

In 1976, eleven Medicaid programs reimbursed skilled-care facilities using Medicare's definition of reasonable cost.[17] Title XVIII defines reasonable cost as "all necessary and proper expenses of an institution in the production of services."[18] These expenses include administrative and maintenance costs as well as the direct and indirect costs of health-care services. To quantify reasonable costs for reimbursement purposes, Medicare has established two methods of calculation.

The first method calculates Medicare's bill by breaking down the total costs of the extended-care institution by divisions, which are distinguished by services produced. For example, the Medicare program reimburses only extended-care facilities in the long-term-care sector and only for 100 days. Medicaid does not recognize extended-care facilities for reimbursement purposes, but extended-care facilities are similar to skilled-care facilities. The number of Medicare patients who use the services of a division is compared to the total number of patients in the institution who utilize these services. This ratio of Medicare users to non-Medicare users is an attempt to measure the amount of resources consumed by Medicare patients. This ratio is then multiplied by the total operating costs for the corresponding division of the facility, which yields Medicare's share of the costs of delivering these services. By summing these divisional charges for all Medicare patients, this method calculates Medicare's share of the total nursing-home costs.

The second method used to calculate the Medicare program's reimbursement costs is a two-step process. In the first step the average per diem cost is calculated for the delivery of routine services for each patient. These routine services are defined by Medicare as room, board, and nursing services. These per diem costs are computed by dividing the total allowable costs for routine services, attributable to Medicare patients, by the total number of Medicare-patient days in an accounting period.

In the second step of this method, the cost of specialized medical treatments is added to the per diem costs for all routine services delivered. These ancillary costs are measured by calculating the ratio of the number of Medicare patients who utilize each specialized treatment to the total number of all patients who receive each of these treatments. Each of these ratios is then multiplied by the total cost of delivery for each of these specialized services to compute Medicare's share of the costs. The sum of all per diem charges for routine services to Medicare patients, combined with Medicare's share of the costs for ancillary services, is the total institution cost of care delivered to Medicare patients for each institution. This reasonable-cost-related method produces a different rate for each institution.

Fixed-Rate Method. With a fixed- or flat-rate-reimbursement method, all long-term-care facilities within the same classification of care are paid the same rate by the Medicaid program. For example, if a state program reimbursed all nursing homes with the fixed-rate method, then all skilled-care facilities would receive an identical flat rate. All intermediate-care facilities would also receive an identical fixed fee, although usually at a lower amount than for skilled care.

If the fixed-rate method is used, the adopting state program determines both the amount and the criteria for setting the rate. In 1975, New Hampshire set its flat rate "in accordance with a predetermined percentage of the most-recent calendar- or fiscal-year per diem cost adjusted in accordance with the inflation factor."[19] In other words, one way to establish a flat rate is to audit the actual cost of delivery, adjust that cost upward for inflation, then set the fixed reimbursement rate at an arbitrary fractional percentage of this audit figure.

Another method for setting the fixed-rate figure relates the flat fee to another reimbursement figure such as that used by Medicare or another Medicaid rate. During 1976 the Medicaid program in the District of Columbia reimbursed intermediate care using a fixed-rate method that was a fractional percentage of the "average per diem rate paid for skilled-nursing facilities. . . ."[20]

Negotiated-Rate Method. According to a report issued by a congressional subcommittee, four state Medicaid programs—Louisiana, Missouri, Oklahoma, and Texas—used the negotiated-rate method to determine reimbursement for skilled-care facilities.[21] The same report listed Massachusetts as reimbursing intermediate-care facilities on a negotiated-rate basis. In an interview, however, a Massachusetts Medicaid official stated that his state program has reimbursed intermediate-care facilities with the reasonable-cost-related method since 1968.

Based on an interview with a Texas Medicaid official, the Texas program does not use a negotiated-rate method for payment purposes nor have they done so for at least six years. The Texas Medicaid program uses what the official called a "fixed prospective rate by class of institution." This program recognizes three classes of long-term care: (1) skilled-nursing care; (2) intermediate-care II (minimum nursing care); and (3) intermediate-care III (moderate nursing care). The fixed rates for each class of care are based upon the historic costs from the previous calendar year. The exact figure is determined by the lower of the two methods. The first method ranks in ascending order the actual costs of all nursing homes participating in the Texas Medicaid program. This method selects as the standard that cost that is in the 75th percentile. The second method takes the mean cost of all Texas nursing homes participating in the Medicaid program and adds 6 percent. Whichever of these two rates is lower is selected as the official fixed reimbursement rate for the Texas program.

The Oklahoma Medicaid program negotiates a flat-fee method for payment to nursing homes. Based on an interview with an Oklahoma Medicaid official, a study was done of the cost of operating a 100-bed facility to establish a base for negotiating. This operating expense is then updated to reflect cost-of-living and wage changes. Negotiations were then conducted between the Oklahoma State Nursing Home Association and Medicaid officials. Different rates were negotiated for the different classes of care within the intermediate-care and skilled-care categories. The different classes are distinguished by variance in personnel, primarily nursing hours.

The Missouri negotiated-rate method is unique in that discussions are between the Division of Family Services and the individual long-term-care facilities. Among the many factors considered by the negotiators are: the average rate paid by private parties, the Veteran's Administration, and other third-party purchasers; per diem rates paid by the Medicare program if the nursing home qualifies under Medicare regulations; rates paid by the Missouri Medicaid program to comparable facilities in the same geographical area; the operating costs of the nursing home; characteristics of the physical plant of the nursing home; and special considerations such as management fees, bond-repayment schedules, and increasing costs due to compliance with federal fire and safety regulations.[22]

This discussion describes the official negotiating process as outlined in the "State Plan under Title XIX of the Social Security Act." In an interview, a Missouri Medicaid official said that "to be honest," not much negotiating actually happened. Negotiations were based on "what the state could pay and the nursing home would accept." The actual negotiating criteria were a review of the long-term-care facility's financial statement and rates paid by Medicaid to other similar institutions in the same geographical area.

The Louisiana negotiating process began when the state legislature appropriated a fixed amount of money for private nursing-home care to be financed through the Medicaid program. Next, according to the Louisiana official interviewed, representatives of the nursing-home industry and the Office of Family Services would negotiate daily rates for the different classes of long-term care. These three classes of care were skilled-nursing care, intermediate-care I (moderate nursing care), and intermediate-care II (low nursing care).

The Louisiana negotiating process was similar to the Oklahoma process for negotiating reimbursement rates. Both processes set fixed rates by class of care, and nursing homes within the same classes of care received the same payment rate. Differing only in the formal process for setting the rate, these state programs had reimbursement methods similar to the fixed-rate method. In Missouri, where negotiations were conducted between Medicaid officials and each individual long-term-care facility, nursing homes delivering similar classes of care could have different payment rates. Again, these payment rates were fixed for each nursing home and did not fluctuate in a time period to reflect cost changes.

Reimbursement Methods versus Goals

How do the methods used by the state Medicaid programs compare to the goals established earlier for a payment mechanism?

Goal 1. The reimbursement method should encourage the efficient delivery of institutional long-term care by creating incentives in the reimbursement method to minimize the costs of delivering care.

Reasonable-Cost-Related Method

The reasonable-cost-related method can be criticized for lacking efficiency incentives. If reimbursement is based on costs incurred, then profit is not necessarily penalized if the long-term-care facility does not minimize costs. If calculated retrospectively, this method does not offer incentives to minimize the costs of delivering services. This reimbursement method also does not encourage innovation to discover new techniques to deliver care at lower costs. Dollar ceilings are often placed on reasonable-cost-reimbursement levels in the attempt to provide some efficiency incentive.

Fixed-Rate Method

A positive relationship exists between the fixed-rate method of payment for long-term care and efficiency incentives. Since the long-term-care facility is paid a specific amount for each classification of care, a strong incentive results to minimize the costs of delivering care in order to increase profits. With the fixed-rate-payment method the difference between the fixed amount paid by the Medicaid program and the actual incurred cost of care is the provider's profit. Also, this method encourages innovation to deliver care by less-expensive methods.

Negotiated-Rate Method

The negotiated-rate method reimburses nursing homes using a fixed, negotiated rate. For this reason the efficiency arguments presented for the fixed-rate method also apply to the negotiated-rate method.

Goal 2. The reimbursement level should encourage the delivery only of those services necessary to increase or maintain the patient's health status. To promote the delivery of quality care, the reimbursement method ideally should include a measure of the effectiveness of care, and payment should be related to that quality measure.

Reasonable-Cost-Related Method

The reasonable-cost-related method does not encourage the delivery of only those services necessary to the individual patient's health status. It encourages the delivery of all services reimbursed by the state Medicaid program, whether or not the patient benefits from utilization. With the reasonable-cost-related method, since all allowable costs are reimbursable, the greater the quantity of services consumed, the higher the Medicaid remuneration level. Again, imposition of a dollar ceiling on payments offsets this incentive for inefficiency to some degree.

   The reasonable-cost-related method is not incompatible with an effectiveness- or quality-of-care measure. Such a measure could be used to either reward or penalize nursing homes by increasing or decreasing reimbursement levels based on readings of the quality-of-care measure. The Michigan Medicaid program, which reimburses long-term-care facilities on a reasonable-cost basis, uses a quality-of-care index to either reward or penalize nursing homes by up to one dollar per patient day.[23]

Fixed-Rate Method

The flat-fee method does encourage the delivery of only those services necessary to the patient's health status. With this method there is no incentive to the long-term-care facility to pad the quantity of services delivered. The profit the nursing home receives is the difference between the fixed payment and the cost of delivering the care, encouraging the delivery of only necessary services to minimize costs.

   As with the reasonable-cost-related method, a quality-of-care index could be used with this reimbursement method to reward or penalize payments based on the index scores.

Negotiated-Rate Method

The efficiency arguments associated with the fixed-rate method also apply to the negotiated-rate method.

Goal 3. The reimbursement method should encourage the delivery of long-term care that is consistent in quality with Medicaid-determined standards.

Reasonable-Cost-Related Method

This reimbursement method lessens the danger that long-term-care facilities would deny needed care to patients. As the nursing home receives payment for the cost of Medicaid-covered services, a positive incentive exists to deliver all the reimbursable health-care services a patient's health status requires. In this respect the reasonable-cost-related method promotes the delivery of quality care. This does not mean, however, that this reimbursement method guarantees that the quality of the services actually delivered will be high, or even that services billed to Medicaid are actually consumed by the patient. The Medicaid program, in its role as purchaser of care, should use a quality-of-care index to monitor the quality of the services actually delivered. Payment to the individual nursing homes should be adjusted to punish or reward quality based on this index.

Fixed-Rate Method

This method provides incentives to long-term-care institutions to reduce the quality of the health care delivered to patients. Again, the nursing home's profit with this method is the difference between the fixed rate and the cost of providing care. An incentive with this reimbursement method is to not only reduce the quantity of services delivered but also to reduce the quality. With this payment method in particular, the Medicaid program has the responsibility to monitor the care delivered to guarantee that adequate health-care services were delivered and that these services were of sufficient quality.

Negotiated-Rate Method

Since negotiated rates are actually fixed rates, the discussion concerning the quality of care and the fixed-rate method applies.

Goal 4. To further encourage the efficient utilization of Medicaid resources and to provide for the delivery of proper care, the state Medicaid programs should reimburse a comprehensive range of long-term-health-care services including alternatives to institutional care.

This goal states that the state Medicaid programs should cover a broad range of long-term-care services. Therefore it relates to coverage rather than to a reimbursement method. All three reimbursement methods could be used to pay for a comprehensive range of long-term-care services. For example, the providers of geriatrics day-care services, which are less costly than institutional care but not universally Medicaid reimbursable, could be reimbursed by either the reasonble-cost-related, fixed-rate, or negotiated-rate methods. The purpose of this reimbursement goal is to expand the Medicaid coverage of long-term-care services to utilize resources more efficiently.

Goal 5. Proprietary long-term-care institutions should be allowed to make a competitive rate of return on investment.

Reasonable-Cost-Related Method

Some state Medicaid programs, which use the reasonable-cost-related method, have adopted the Medicare program's profit formula. This formula provides a profit to proprietary long-term-care facilities by recognizing a return on net capital equity as part of the institution's reasonable cost. A fixed percentage of net capital equity becomes reimbursable as a cost of delivering care. The purpose is to provide an incentive to attract capital into the nursing-home industry. This guaranteed profit, however, does not promote efficiency. In fact, basing profit on capital investment provides an incentive to nursing homes to become more capital intensive than is economically efficient or optimal.[24] This reimbursement method distorts decision making on the capital/labor mix to the detriment of minimizing costs.

Fixed-Rate Method

The fixed-rate method can adversely affect profits if the reimbursement-rate figure is set unrealistically low. One danger of an inadequate fixed rate is the incentive it provides to nursing homes to restrict the quantity and quality of services delivered, thereby adversely affecting the quality of care received. Another danger of too low a fixed rate is that proprietary nursing homes would refuse to participate in the Medicaid program. Beverly Enterprises, a for-profit long-term-care chain, plans to limit the number of Medicaid patients it admits in order to increase the number of private patients "who can pay $3-5 more per day. . . ."[25]

Negotiated-Rate Method

If payment rates offered by the Medicaid program in the negotiating process are too low, nursing homes could refuse to participate in the Medicaid program, or they could participate and deliver lower-quality care to Medicaid patients. The arguments are again similar to those directed at the fixed-rate method.

To summarize, the fixed-rate method, with qualifications, fulfills the goals of a reimbursement system better than the reasonable-cost-related method. The fixed-rate method is strongest in the areas of providing incentives for cost reduction by encouraging only the delivery of necessary services and at a minimum cost. In contrast, the reasonable-cost-related method encourages the delivery of all allowable services with no incentives to minimize costs. The use of a reimbursement ceiling somewhat offsets these disincentives to efficiency.

The major potential problem with the fixed-rate method is its negative quality-of-care incentive. To guarantee the quality of care to long-term-care patients is a problem regardless of the payment method used, but the fixed-rate method accentuates the danger. The long-term-care patient/consumer cannot guarantee the quality of care received for economic as well as health-related reasons. Given the incentive to decrease costs to increase profits, the use of a fixed-rate method could result in the delivery of fewer and lower-quality services. The fixed-rate reimbursement level must be sufficiently high to financially allow the delivery of adequate care. The Medicaid program must monitor this care to guarantee that quality care is in fact delivered to patients. A fixed-rate payment method, modified to include a quality-of-care index linking payment levels to the quality of care delivered, may be the reimbursement method to harness the profit motive to promote efficiency and to protect against patient abuse in the delivery of long-term care.

Reimbursement Experiments

In addition to the need to control the rising costs of the Medicare and Medicaid programs, the increased possibility of a national health-insurance plan increases the need to experiment in order to discover efficiency incentives in reimbursement methods. A possibility, however, with any efficiency-incentive features in a reimbursement method is the danger that cost cutting could adversely affect the quality of care and hence patient health levels.

One approach to this problem is to encourage research that links health-care services consumed by patients with changes in patient health levels. State health departments, for example, could be encouraged to undertake this research in their states through the federal grant system. If medical research can establish which long-term-care services have the greatest impact on patient health in the various classifications of care, then quality of care can be guaranteed by mandating the delivery of these essential health services through Medicaid requirements for certification. The Medicaid program can monitor nursing homes with a quality-of-care index to assure delivery and base reimbursement upon the index score. With quality controlled, the danger that cost cutting, encouraged by efficiency incentives in the reimbursement method, would adversely affect health levels is decreased.

Incentive Reimbursement Method

Ruchlin, Levey, and Muller have proposed an incentive reimbursement model.[26] They argue that per diem reimbursement should be a function of four factors: (1) facility grouping and the establishment of dollar ceilings within each group; (2) degree of resource utilization (occupancy rates); (3) patient assessment and classification into health-status categories; and (4) facility evaluation.[27]

Facility Grouping. Five criteria are proposed to determine facility classification: (1) facility type including hospital type, other institution, or ambulatory-care services; (2) size of facility; (3) geographical location—whether central city, noncentral city, or rural; (4) type of ownership; and (5) whether hospital affiliated or not.

A preliminary per diem reimbursement rate would be set based upon the average per diem cost of all nursing homes within each classification grouping. According to this proposed payment model, a specified ceiling would be set above this group average. Reimbursement above the average, and up to the ceiling, would only be allowed if the institution could document to the Medicaid program that these costs above the group mean resulted from the provision of quality-improvement-related services.

Occupancy Rates. A minimum occupancy rate would be established under this proposed reimbursement model for each classification of nursing-home groupings. If occupancy rates for an institution fell below the minimum rate, the per diem reimbursement the nursing home received would be adjusted downward. The purpose of the adjustment is to apply pressure on the long-term-care facility to improve its operating efficiency.

Patient Assessment and Classification. Patients within a nursing home would be subjected to annual medical/social/behavioral evaluations to develop a patient-health-status index (PHSI) for each facility. The PHSI for each nursing home would be compared to the average of all other institutions within the same classification. This comparison would determine the intensity of patient care each long-term-care facility delivers relative to other nursing homes in the same category. A long-term-care institution with a relatively higher PHSI would have its average per diem reimbursement rate adjusted upward from the group mean.

Facility Evaluation. To qualify for participation in the Medicaid program, this proposed reimbursement system would require that all nursing homes be evaluated by an appropriate government agency. This evaluation would certify, if successful, that a nursing home was eligible to deliver care and receive Medicaid payments.

This model compares favorably with the goals established for reimbursement methods. Reimbursement is at a fixed rate for each classification grouping and is based on the average cost of delivering care within that group. This payment model puts pressure on long-term-care facilities to deliver care below this average total cost by delivering only necessary services at a minimum cost if the institutions want to earn a profit. The model does encourage the delivery of quality care because of the facility-evaluation aspect. Also, quality care is encouraged because the nursing home can be reimbursed above the average per diem cost if the facility can document that the care was necessary to improve quality. Finally, this model encourages the delivery of quality care because the payment rate is adjusted upward to reflect increased patient-health needs based upon the PHSI.

The Johns Hopkins Experiment

An interesting reimbursement experiment is the project agreement between the Maryland Medicaid program and Johns Hopkins Hospital.[28] Under the terms of the agreement, Johns Hopkins provides Medicaid-covered services to up to 3,500 Medicaid-eligible patients for a per capita payment of $23.55 per month. An additional $10 per capita payment is made for use in meeting start-up costs.

If the plan's costs are less than the monthly per capita payments, the hospital receives a payment of 50 percent of the difference as an incentive. If the costs exceed payments, the plan will reimburse the hospital to cover the cost overruns. However, the unique feature of the plan is that any future incentive payments will be reduced by as much as 50 percent to offset past cost overruns.

By allowing Johns Hopkins to recover all cost overruns, needed medical services will not have to be sacrificed to lower costs. However, adjusting future incentive reimbursements to recover past cost overruns provides the stimulus to minimize present operating costs. This is an interesting aspect of the Johns Hopkins/Maryland Medicaid reimbursement experiment and should be considered in all incentive reimbursement programs.

This experiment could easily be adapted to reimburse nursing-home care. Long-term-care patients could be classified according to the PHSI and then placed into health-status categories based upon their PHSI. A fixed, monthly reimbursement rate would then be assigned to each health-status classification.

If the nursing home's costs are less than the monthly per capita payments, then the long-term-care facility would receive a payment of 50 percent of the difference as an efficiency reward. If the actual incurred costs exceed the monthly payment, then the nursing home would be reimbursed to cover the overruns. Future incentive payments would be adjusted to offset past cost overruns.

This proposed reimbursement method compares favorably with the goals for a reimbursement method. By allowing the long-term-care facility to retain 50 percent of any cost savings, an incentive is provided to minimize the costs of care, with both the Medicaid program and the nursing home receiving the financial benefits.

By reimbursing the long-term-care facility for cost overruns, the patient's health status is not sacrificed to cost cutting. Yet reductions of future cost savings to repay these overruns provide an incentive to the nursing home to minimize overruns. This proposed method allows the long-term-care institution to benefit from its efficiency by permitting the facility to retain as profit 50 percent of the cost savings.

Prospective- and Retrospective-Rate Determination

Another long-term-care reimbursement issue relates to prospective- versus retrospective-rate determination.[29] Traditionally, most state Medicaid payments for nursing-home care have been established retrospectively—that is, costs are determined at the end of the applicable time period. The payment by the Medicaid program to the long-term-care institution is adjusted to cover the actual incurred costs to the health-care provider of delivering reimbursable services. Some state Medicaid programs have placed an upper limit on the amount of retrospective per diem patient costs. The distinctive feature of retrospective reimbursement is the retroactive determination of costs for reimbursement.

The distinctive feature of prospective reimbursement is that the payment rate is established prior to the period the rate is to be applied.[30] Nursing homes must deliver long-term care at the predetermined rate. If the actual delivery cost is above the prospective rate, then the nursing home must absorb all or a portion of these cost overruns, depending on the particular regulations of the states' Medicaid programs. Conversely, the nursing home is allowed to keep all or a portion of any excess of the prospective rate over the actual delivery costs as an incentive toward increased efficiency.[31]

Table 3-1 summarizes the past use of prospective and retrospective reimbursement. (See appendix C for a listing of these states.)

Either the prospective or retrospective method can be used in conjunction with reasonable-cost-related reimbursement, fixed-rate reimbursement, or negotiated-rate reimbursement. State Medicaid programs using the reasonable-cost-related method can calculate its per diem rate either prospectively or retrospectively. The negotiated-rate and fixed-rate methods of reimbursement are typically associated with the prospective method. However, not all states using either the fixed-rate or the negotiated-rate methods determine their rates on a strictly prospective basis. During 1977, for example, Michigan used the fixed-rate method to reimburse for skilled care (see appendix I). This Medicaid program also calculated its rate retrospectively (see appendix C). The explanation is that the Michigan program allows the retroactive readjustment of its fixed-rate payment.

In a time of inflation, retrospective reimbursement is clearly to the advantage of the health-care providers because it assures full payment for the costs of allowable services delivered. This type of reimbursement may also be indirectly advantageous to the patients in long-term-care institutions in that needed medical care will not be sacrificed to cost cutting. However, this assurance of full-cost payment with retrospective reimbursement is a two-edged sword. Payment to nursing homes based on the retrospective calculation of the full costs of providing care is completely lacking in incentives for efficiency and cost control—this is the major weakness of this type of reimbursement mechanism. According to one study, the impact of retrospective rate setting has been to offer health-care providers the opportunity to add new personnel and equipment, to raise wages, and to expand services and facilities with the knowledge that any cost increases will be passed along as part of the patient's bill.[32] This potential for inefficiency in retrospective reimbursement can be reduced by establishing ceilings on retrospective payments. Payment ceilings do not provide incentives for cost cutting and efficiency, however, as much as they place an upper limit on an acceptable level of inefficiency.

The major argument for prospective reimbursement is that it will

Table 3–1
The Number of States Using Prospective- and Retrospective-Rate
Determination

Year	Prospective		Retrospective	
	Skilled Care	Intermediate Care	Skilled Care	Intermediate Care
1977	24	26	19	17
1976	19	21	17	15
1975	15	15	24	24

provide needed incentives for cost containment. Since payment rates are established in advance, the administrators of long-term-care facilities must deliver the prescribed level of care at a cost below the prospective rate if they want to make a profit. The prospective method removes from the state Medicaid programs the burden of increased costs caused by inefficiency and mismanagement and properly places it with the nursing-home administrators.[33] Prospective payments encourage long-term-care administrators to develop management techniques to monitor and control costs. Based on these efficiency incentives, a study of long-term-care reimbursement by consultants for the DHHS endorsed prospective reimbursement as "the superior alternative" to retrospective-rate setting.[34]

In times of a virulent inflationary spiral as experienced during the 1970s, the prospective-rate-setting method offers the greatest promise of controlling health-care costs. As rates are set in advance, the administrators of long-term-care facilities cannot easily pass along cost increases to the Medicaid program. As mentioned before, the prospective method places the burden of cost inefficiencies and increases on the nursing home, not the state Medicaid programs. Contrary to the effect of retrospective reimbursement, which can add to the inflationary spiral by passing along cost increases to the Medicaid program with no attempt to decrease costs, the prospective system can help fight inflation in the health-care segment of the U.S. economy by providing incentives to nursing-home operators to innovate to reduce costs.

Other supporters of prospective reimbursement include (not surprisingly) state Medicaid and Blue Cross administrators. Blue Cross of Rhode Island estimated it saved $9.8 million on acute hospital-care expenditures in fiscal years 1976 and 1977 through the use of prospective reimbursement. According to Raymond Caine, a vice-president of the plan, "The days are gone when a hospital can just spend money and pass the costs along to the third-party payer."[35]

A University of Washington study estimated that the use of prospective reimbursement in New York State saved the Medicaid and Blue Cross programs $51 million a year between 1970 and 1974 in downstate acute-care-hospital payments alone.[36] During 1977 the New York Medicaid program expected payments for in-hospital care to be about $935 million, up less than 2 percent from the year before, with a savings of $65 million attributed to its use of prospective reimbursement.[37]

Prospective reimbursement is not without its critics, however. For example, after St. Luke's Hospital was exposed to the prospective-payment method used by the New York State Medicaid program, the hospital's vice-president for administration lamented in reference to the state's effort to squeeze fat from his hospital's operations: "We wonder if the state knows the difference between a squeeze and a stranglehold."[38] St. Luke's accumulated an operating deficit of more than $16 million between 1970 and 1975 due to prospective reimbursement.

The possibility exists that unrealistically low prospective rates will force health-care providers to cut the quality of services and treatments to maintain financial viability. With the increased use of prospective reimbursement, state Medicaid programs have the increased responsibility to assure that the payment rate is sufficient to provide for needed high-quality care and that health-care providers will not reduce needed services to minimize costs to increase profits. This potential threat to the quality of the health care delivered is an inherent problem with the prospective-reimbursement method.

In addition to the threats to the quality of care, another danger exists to the long-term-care-delivery system if the prospective-reimbursement rate is set too low—that is, nursing-home corporations may refuse to participate in the Medicaid program. If the prospective rate set by state Medicaid programs is not comparable to private rates, then finding available beds for Medicaid patients requiring long-term care may become difficult.

One other potential problem with prospective reimbursement warrants mention. Critics have charged that when prospective reimbursement is used to pay for acute hospital care, hospitals attempt to offset the lower limits of per diem payments by keeping the patients for longer stays. In other words, hospitals stretch out the length of stay to increase revenues in order to overcome lower per diem payments.[39] Does this charge against prospective reimbursement for hospital care also apply to prospective reimbursement for long-term care?

Advocates of prospective reimbursement have claimed this this payment method encourages efficiency in the delivery of health-care services and holds down cost increases. In the area of long-term-care delivery, does prospective reimbursement encourage cost containment? Are per diem reimbursement rates established by the prospective method lower than retrospective per diem rates? Are there significant differences in the rate of cost increases between these two methods?

Critics of prospective reimbursement have claimed that this payment method affects the utilization of care. Does prospective reimbursement have a negative impact on the utilization of long-term care by Medicaid patients? In states that utilize the prospective method, are fewer Medicaid patients receiving nursing-home care? Do those Medicaid patients admitted stay longer to increase total per-patient revenues?

In the next chapter cost and utilization indexes are developed in an attempt to answer these questions. These measures will then be applied to the national long-term-health-care system to assess what impact prospective and retrospective reimbursement have had on the cost and utilization of nursing-home care.

Notes

1. M. Keith Weikel and Nancy Leamond, "A Decade of Medicaid," *Public Health Reports* 91 (July–August 1976):304.

2. Ibid.

3. Ibid.

4. U.S., Department of Health, Education, and Welfare, Comptroller General of the United States, "Problems in Providing Guidance to the States in Estimating Rates of Payment for NHC under Medicaid Program," *Social and Rehabilitative Services,* 19 April 1972, p. 5.

5. "Entitlement to Hospital Insurance Benefits," *The United States Code,* vol. 9, sec. 426, p. 9857 (1970).

6. Department of Health, Education, and Welfare, "Problems in Providing Guidance," pp. 5-6.

7. U.S., *Statutes at Large,* vol. 85, p. 809.

8. U.S., Department of Health, Education, and Welfare, *National Center for Health Statistics 1975,* DHEW Publication, no. HRA 76:1232, (1976).

9. Weikel and Leamond, "A Decade of Medicaid," p. 307.

10. "States Put Scalpel to Medicaid in Budget-Cutting Operation," *National Journal* 8 (1 May 1976):581.

11. *National Journal* 7 (7 September 1975):1319.

12. *National Journal* 8 (1 May 1976):583.

13. Ibid.

14. Paul Ginsberg, "Cost Containment Through Reforming Nursing-Home Reimbursement," in *Academe and State Legislative Policies for Health,* ed. Selma Mushkin (Washington, D.C.: Public Services Laboratory, Georgetown University, December 1976), p. 25.

15. Hirsch Ruchlin, Samuel Levey, and Charlotte Muller, "The Long-Term Care Marketplace," *Medical Care* 13:982.

16. Ginsberg, "Cost Containment Through Reform," p. 26.

17. U.S., Congress, House of Representatives Interstate and Foreign Commerce Committee, *Data on the Medicaid Program,* 95th Congress, 1st Sess., 1977, pp. 20–21.

18. U.S., Department of Health, Education, and Welfare, Social Security Administration, *Principles of Reimbursement for Provider Costs,* USDHEW, HIM-5, January 1967, citing Public Law 89–97, p. 1.

19. U.S., Department of Health, Education, and Welfare, Health Care Finance Administration, "State Plan under Title XIX of the Social Security Act," *Methods and Standards for Establishing Payment Rates,* Medical Assistance Program, DHEW, OPC-11, 75–17; Attachment 4.19.B, State of New Hampshire, p. 2.

20. U.S., Health Care Finance Administration, ibid., District of Columbia, p. 3.

21. Interstate and Foreign Commerce Committee, *Data on the Medicaid Program,* p. 20.

22. U.S., Health Care Finance Administration, "State Plan under Title XIX," Missouri, p. 10.

23. Ibid., Michigan, p. 2.

24. Harvey Averech and LeLand Johnson, "Behavior of the Firm under Regulatory Constraint, *American Economic Review* 52 (December 1962):1052–1069.

25. "Nursing the Nursing Homes," *Business Week* 5 December 1977, p. 70.

26. Ruchlin, Levey, Muller, "Long-Term Care Marketplace," pp. 979–91.

27. Ibid., p. 982.

28. Glenn Martin, "Incentives for Economy," *Hospitals,* 1 October 1971, p. 54.

29. Applied Management Sciences, *Report on Systems of Reimbursement for Long-Term Care: vol. I: Analyses and Recommendations,* 7 April 1976, pp. 2.1–2.9.

30. John Inglehart, "Government Searching for a More Cost-Efficient Way to Pay for Hospitals, *National Journal* (25 December 1976):1822–29.

31. Applied Management Sciences, *Report on Systems of Reimbursement,* p. 2.1.

32. Katherine Bauer, "Containing Cost of Health Services Through Incentive Reimbursement," in *Report on Systems of Reimbursement for Long-Term Care,* Applied Management Sciences, p. 2.2.

33. Ibid.

34. Ibid., p. 2.4.

35. Jeffrey Tannenbaum, "Medical Squeeze," *Wall Street Journal,* 21 June 1977, p. 1.

36. Ibid., p. 35.

37. Ibid.

38. Ibid., p. 1.

39. Ibid., p. 35.

Cost and Utilization Analysis of the Reimbursement Methods

Statistical Tools

Two related statistical techniques—difference of means and analysis of variance—were used in the attempt to determine whether differences in reimbursement methods have had an impact on the delivery of nursing-home care.[1]

Difference of Means

The difference-of-means test calculates a ratio in which the numerator measures the differences between two group means, and the denominator measures the variability of individual outcomes around their groups means for each of the two groups. This ratio is expressed as either a Z or a T score. The T score is used when the number of observations in each group is less than thirty. The larger the difference between the two group means (the numerator) in relation to the difference within groups (the denominator), the larger the T or Z score.

A difference-of-means test is used when a comparison between two group means is required. Difference-of-means tests were used in this study to determine whether significant differences existed between the group of states that determined their payment rates prospectively and the group of states that used the retrospective method for cost and utilization variables.

Analysis of Variance

Analysis of variance is a concept related to the difference-of-means test, but it is used when three or more groups are to be compared. It is a technique that, like difference of means, compares the amount of variation in outcomes *among* groups against the variation among outcomes *within* groups. Analysis of variance was used in this study to determine whether a significant difference existed among states using different reimbursement methods for cost and utilization variables.

As the name implies, analysis of variance is concerned with the variation of observed outcomes. This variation is expressed in an F ratio. The

49

numerator of this ratio measures the distance of group means from one another and is referred to as the variation among groups. The denominator measures the distance of outcomes from their group mean and is referred to as the variation within groups. The larger the difference among groups (the numerator) in relation to the variations within groups (the denominator), the larger the F score.

The Z and T scores are the expression of the ratio of the difference-of-means test. The F score is the expression of the ratio of the analysis of variance. These ratios are an expression of the variation among groups compared to the variation within groups. These Z, T, and F scores are important because the larger the ratio of among-group variation compared to within-group variation, the greater the probability that statistically significant differences exist among the groups. A statistically significant difference is defined as a difference among groups that is attributed to population differences and not to random events.[2] In statistical analysis the size of the Z, T, or F score enables the analyst to either reject or accept the null hypothesis.

Null Hypothesis

The null hypothesis states that the groups in question are not really distinct, separate populations but actually subgroups from a single population. In other words, the null hypothesis states that no difference exists among groups for the variables in question. For example, the null hypothesis states that the means of average per diem costs for the different reimbursement methods do not differ because for the variable in question these reimbursement methods are really only subgroups of the same populations, not separate populations. Separate populations would statistically imply that the reimbursement method had an impact on the variable in question—the average per diem cost, for example.

If a sufficiently greater difference exists between groups than variability within groups, which the Z, T, and F scores measure, then the null hypothesis can be rejected. It is then assumed that a statistically significant difference exists among reimbursement methods for the dependent variable in question. The conclusion in this study would be that the reimbursement method has an effect, or impact, on the variable in question.

The null hypothesis of this analysis is that the groupings of the different reimbursement methods are subgroups of one single population and that the reimbursement methods have no impact on the dependent variable. The statistical analysis reveals whether the null hypothesis can be rejected or not. If the null hypothesis is rejected, it is assumed that the different reimbursement practices are separate populations and not subgroups of the same populations. This in turn means, from a statistical perspective, that reimbursement methods do affect the dependent variables used in the study. These dependent variables are: Medicaid patients per 1,000 elderly, Medicaid patients days per 1,000 elderly, average length of stay, average per diem cost, and average annual per diem–cost increases. These dependent variables are analyzed separately for skilled and intermediate care.

Level of Significance

The level of significance is a critical issue in statistical analysis because it is what determines how large a Z, T, or F score is required in order to reject the null hypothesis. The level of significance determines what degree of risk the analyst is willing to accept of rejecting a null hypothesis that should in fact not be rejected. The larger the Z, T, or F score, the less likely a researcher will make an error by rejecting the null hypothesis that in reality is correct. The level of significance is the standard or benchmark set by researchers to guide them in accepting or rejecting a null hypothesis.

As a matter of convention, many social scientists use .05 as their level of significance to guide them in their decisions on null-hypothesis rejection. This means that researchers are willing to reject the null hypothesis if the observed differences between group means could occur by chance only 5 times or less out of every 100 occurrences. They are willing to assume that differences between the observed group means are attributable to population differences and not to random events if there is only a 5-in-100 probability that chance could generate the observed group means.

Nothing is sacred, however, about the .05 significance level. Other levels such as .01 have also been used by statisticians. The lower the significance level selected, the less danger there is in rejecting a null hypothesis that should be accepted. In statistical terms this danger is known as an alpha or Type-I error. If a significance level of .01 is selected, and the Z, T, or F ratio is sufficiently large to reject the null hypothesis, then the probability that random events could generate the observed group means is 1 out of 100 or less. With a level of significance this low, the probability of committing an alpha error is extremely small.

Using a significance level of .01, or any low level of significance, presents the danger of not rejecting a null hypothesis that in fact should be rejected. This potential danger is known statistically as a beta or Type-II error. To minimize the possibility of an alpha error requires a low level of significance. Conversely, to minimize the possibility of a beta error requires a higher level of significance. Selecting the level of significance for any statistical analysis requires a tradeoff—that is, to reduce the probability of an alpha error the researcher increases the probability of a beta error. The converse is also true.

One social scientist has suggested that if the researcher is "exploring a set of relationships'' for the purpose of developing hypotheses, then a significance level of .10 or .20 would be acceptable.[3] These relatively high levels of significance would reduce the chances of committing a beta error—accepting a null hypothesis that should be rejected. Since the null hypothesis always assumes no difference between groups, a .10 level of significance would yield more working hypotheses that the groups actually do differ than would a .05 significance level. Since the .10 or .20 significance level was recommended for exploratory research, the purpose of which is to develop hypotheses about relationships rather than to state conclusions, the increased probability of committing an alpha error is acceptable. Since this analysis is exploring the relationships between reimbursement methods and cost and utilization measures, a .10 significance level has been selected.

To summarize the statistical methodology, the tools of difference of means and analysis of variance were used in this study. These tests generated F or T ratios that compare the variability among groups to the variability within groups. These ratios are used either to accept or reject the null hypothesis. In this analysis the null hypothesis states that no difference exists in the cost and utilization means among the different reimbursement methods. The null hypothesis states that the groupings by different reimbursement methods are not separate, distinct populations, but subgroups of the same population. If the F or T ratios are sufficiently large to permit rejection of the null hypothesis, then this indicates that statistically significant differences exist for the means of the different cost and utilization measures among reimbursement methods. This in turn indicates that the reimbursement method has an impact on the dependent variable in question. (For a difference among means to be statistically significant states that the observed difference among reimbursement methods can be attributed to population differences and not to chance.)

The level of significance chosen to determine whether the null hypotheses should be accepted or rejected is .10 or less. If the null hypothesis is rejected, then there is 1 chance in 10 or less that the observed differences among means for the dependent variables occurred due to chance and not because of population differences. The actual level of significance, however, is reported in the text. These reported significance levels state the probability of the observed differences among reimbursement methods occurring by chance rather than due to population differences.

Cost and Utilization Measures

The central question of this analysis is whether the different reimbursement practices used by state Medicaid programs affect the cost and utilization of long-term care. Do reasonable-cost-related reimbursement, fixed-rate reimbursement, negotiated-rate reimbursement, and prospective- and retrospective-rate determination affect the cost of nursing-home care to the state Medicaid programs? Do these reimbursement techniques influence how the elderly Medicaid patients utilize long-term care? This analysis has developed cost and utilization measures to assess these impacts.

Cost Measures

The primary cost measure used in this study is the average per diem rate used by state Medicaid programs to reimburse for the different types of long-term care. Do the means of the average per diem costs for the different reimbursement methods differ significantly? If so, which reimbursement method has the lower average per diem cost?

This cost measure is an attempt to determine if any of the reimbursement methods encourage cost containment in the delivery of nursing-home care. The basic assumption is that the quality of care does not differ between reimbursement methods. If one payment method encouraged the delivery of care at a lower cost, but of a lower quality, then this method of payment would not encourage more-efficient delivery of care; it would encourage only the delivery of less-expensive care. Since assessing the quality of care is beyond the scope of this study, this analysis can only answer the question: Do reimbursement methods affect the price of care? Per diem cost is a proxy measure for efficiency in this study.

The other cost measure used in this study is the average annual cost increase. Are there statistically significant differences in annual cost increases among the different reimbursement methods? Since Medicaid expenditures for long-term care are increasing annually at a dramatic rate, this becomes an important question. What are the differences, if any, in cost increases between the different payment methods?

Utilization Measures

Utilization measures are an attempt to determine whether reimbursement affects the consumption pattern of long-term care by Medicaid patients. Do the methods of reimbursement used by state Medicaid programs affect the availability of nursing-home care to Medicaid patients? Do the different reimbursement methods affect the attractiveness of Medicaid patients to the long-term-care industry?

The number of Medicaid patients receiving each type of long-term care per 1,000 of each state's elderly population was one utilization measure developed (see appendixes D and E). This indicator measures the number of elderly Medicaid patients receiving each type of nursing-home care in each state. Placing this figure in a ratio of per-1,000 elderly controls for population variances among states. A similar measure developed was the number of Medicaid patient days per 1,000 of each state's elderly population (see appendixes F and G). These indicators are attempts to measure the impact different reimbursement methods have on the willingness of the nursing-home industry to accept Medicaid patients.

Critics of prospective-rate determination have claimed that this reimbursement method encourages acute-care hospitals to stretch out patients' stays to increase per-patient revenues. Do the different long-term-care-reimbursement practices affect the length of patient stay? The average length of stay was the utilization measure used to answer this question (see appendix H).

These cost and utilization indicators were developed to measure the impact, if any, that Medicaid reimbursement has had on the delivery of nursing-home care. These indicators are the dependent variables of this analysis. The study focuses on a five-year period from 1973 to 1977, the latter being the most-recent year for which data is available. In addition to the annual breakdown of the analysis, comparisons were made separately for skilled care and intermediate care (see appendix I).

Prospective- versus Retrospective-Rate Determination

In retrospective-rate setting the state Medicaid programs retroactively adjust payments to nursing homes to reflect the actual cost of delivering the care. The distinctive feature of prospective reimbursement is the fact that the payment is established prior to the period to which the rate is applied. Do these two different methods for calculating payments affect the cost of care to the Medicaid program and the utilization of care by Medicaid patients?

Limited data are available from the states on the use of prospective- and retrospective-rate setting. Telephone interviews with state Medicaid officials and a mail survey generated data on which states used prospective and which used retrospective payments in 1977 and 1976. A study by Applied Management Sciences revealed the data for 1975.[4] The data needed to develop this study's utilization measures for 1977 and beyond were not available from the Department of Health and Human Services at the time of this research. Therefore, the utilization analysis for prospective- and retrospective-rate calculation is only for the years 1975 and 1976. The cost analysis is for 1975 through 1977.

Utilization Indexes

Does a statistically significant difference exist between the prospective and retrospective methods for the number of Medicaid patients (65 and over) per 1,000 of each state's population (65 and over)? This analysis is an attempt to determine whether these different methods for setting payment rates affect the willingness of the long-term-care industry to accept Medicaid patients. The null hypothesis declares that the states grouped together according to prospective- and retrospective-rate determination are not really separate populations but actually subgroups of the same population. No difference is evident for the averages of the different utilization indicators between prospective and retrospective reimbursement. The impact of these two rate-setting methods are presented first for skilled care and then for intermediate care.

Skilled Care.

Medicaid Patients. For neither 1975 nor 1976 can the null hypothesis be rejected. No statistically significant difference exists between the rate-setting methods for the average number of Medicaid patients receiving skilled care per 1,000 elderly (see table 4–1). Prospective and retrospective reimbursement do not affect the number of Medicaid patients receiving skilled care in nursing homes. During 1976 states using prospective reimbursement averaged 13.7 skilled-care patients per 1,000 of each state's elderly population. States using the retrospective method averaged 16.2 patients per 1,000 of their elderly population. According to the statistical analysis, these observed outcomes could occur by chance 60 out of every 100 times. During 1975 states using prospective reimbursement had more patients per 1,000 elderly of their population receiving skilled care, which was the opposite from the 1976 results. Statistical analysis reveals a high probability that differences between prospective and retrospective reimbursement for the average number of skilled-care patients per 1,000 elderly are due to chance and not population differences.

Table 4–1
Medicaid Patients (Aged 65 and over) per 1,000 Elderly—Skilled Care

Year	Prospective	Retrospective	Level of Significance
1976	13.7	16.2	0.60
1975	20.6	16.8	0.47

Table 4-2
Medicaid Patient Days (Aged 65 and over) per 1,000 Elderly—Skilled Care

Year	Prospective	Retrospective	Level of Significance
1976	2,833	2,840	0.99
1975	4,275	3,233	0.35

Medicaid Patient Days. For neither 1975 nor 1976 can the null hypothesis be rejected. No statistically significant difference exists between the rate-setting methods for the average number of Medicaid patient days of skilled care per 1,000 elderly (see table 4-2). Prospective and retrospective reimbursement does not affect the average number of Medicaid patient days of skilled care per 1,000 elderly population. There is also no consistency in the observed differences for the two years. During 1976 states using retrospective reimbursement had the higher average; during 1975 states using prospective reimbursement had the higher average. To interpret the statistical meaning of these findings, during 1976 the observed differences between prospective- and retrospective-rate setting for this utilization index could have occurred by chance 99 out of every 100 times.

Average Length of Stay. Prospective and retrospective reimbursements do not affect the average length of stay of Medicaid patients at skilled-care facilities (see table 4-3).

In the case of the delivery of acute hospital care, critics of prospective-rate determination have charged that hospitals will stretch out the length of stay for patients whose care is financed through prospective payments to increase per-patient revenues. This does not appear to be the case for Medicaid patients receiving skilled care financed with prospective-reimbursement payments. During 1976 the average length of stay for skilled-care patients in states using prospective reimbursement was 147 days. In states using retrospective reimbursement, the average for this utilization measure was also 147 days. During 1975 the average length of stay for skilled-care patients in states using the prospective method was 189 days, longer than the 156-day average for states using the retrospective method. The difference, however, was not statistically significant. This observed outcome could occur by chance 17 out of every 100 times. Given the .10 level of significance, the probability that chance affected the outcome is too high to reject the null hypothesis.

Summary. To summarize the effect of prospective and retrospective reimbursement on the utilization indexes for skilled-care patients, the null hypo-

Table 4-3
Average Length of Stay (Prospective and Retrospective) for Medicaid Patients—Skilled Care

Year	Prospective	Retrospective	Level of Significance
1976	147	147	0.99
1975	189	156	0.17

Table 4-4
Medicaid Patients (Aged 65 and over) per 1,000 Elderly—Intermediate Care

Year	Prospective	Retrospective	Level of Significance
1976	29.8	23.6	0.18
1975	16.6	23.5	0.09

thesis cannot be rejected in any instance. Prospective- and retrospective-rate determinations do not affect the number of skilled-care patients per 1,000 elderly, the number of skilled-care patient days per 1,000 elderly, or the average length of stay. The use of prospective reimbursement did not discourage long-term-care institutions from accepting skilled-care patients during 1975 and 1976. Based on the findings of this analysis, apparently none of the criticisms of prospective reimbursement in terms of a negative impact on access to skilled care by Medicaid patients is warranted.

Intermediate Care.

Medicaid Patients. The difference between rate-setting methods for the average number of Medicaid patients receiving intermediate care per 1,000 elderly population is significant for 1975 (see table 4-4). States that used retrospective-rate determination had the higher average number of inter-mediate-care patients per 1,000 elderly. For this year the null hypothesis can be rejected, meaning that in 1975 prospective- and retrospective-rate setting seemed to affect the number of Medicaid patients receiving intermediate care.

Somewhat offsetting this conclusion, however, is the fact that in 1976 states that used the prospective method had the higher average for this measure, reversing the results from the previous year. The difference in 1976, however, was not statistically significant. This inconsistency between

the two years for the average number of Medicaid patients receiving intermediate care per 1,000 elderly population qualifies the conclusion for 1975.

Medicaid Patient Days. The difference between rate-setting methods for
the average number of Medicaid patient days of intermediate care per 1,000
elederly is not significant for the years 1975 and 1976 (see table 4–5). There
is also no consistency in the observed averages. During 1975 states using the
retrospective method of rate setting had the higher reading for this utilization measure. During 1976 states using the prospective method had the
higher average.

Average Length of Stay. The average length of stay for Medicaid patients
receiving intermediate care in nursing homes does not differ, from a statistical perspective, among states using prospective and retrospective reimbursement (see table 4–6). In neither year can the null hypothesis be rejected
for the average length-of-stay index.

Summary. To summarize the impact of prospective and retrospective reimbursement during 1975 and 1976 on the utilization indexes for intermediate
care, no statistically significant difference existed in the averages for the
utilization measures between the two methods for setting payment rates. In
only one instance could the null hypothesis be rejected. During 1975 a statistically significant greater number of patients received intermediate care in
states using the retrospective method than in states using the prospective
method. However, this difference was offset when the reverse outcome
occurred the next year for this utilization measure.

Utilization Conclusions

In the utilization of both intermediate and skilled care, apparently prospec-
tive- and retrospective-rate determination have had no impact. The use of
prospective reimbursement did not discourage nursing homes from accepting Medicaid patients when compared to states using retrospective reimbursement during the two years analyzed. The use of prospective reimbursement did not encourage long-term-care facilities to increase the length
of stay by Medicaid patients in order to increase per-patient revenues. The
potential dangers that nursing homes would refuse to accept Medicaid
patients in states using prospective reimbursement, and stretch out the
length of stay for those accepted, did not occur during 1976 and 1975 based
on the findings of this study. However, did the touted cost savings attributed to prospective-rate determination occur?

Table 4-5
Medicaid Patient Days (Aged 65 and over) per 1,000 Elderly—Intermediate Care

Year	Prospective	Retrospective	Level of Significance
1976	7,298	5,124	0.11
1975	3,953	5,530	0.13

Table 4-6
Average Length of Stay (Prospective and Retrospective) for Medicaid Patients—Intermediate Care

Year	Prospective	Retrospective	Level of Significance
1976	243	219	0.12
1975	226	225	0.94

Cost Indexes

Does prospective-rate setting encourage cost containment in the delivery of long-term care? Does a difference exist in the average per diem price paid for long-term care among states using prospective and retrospective reimbursement?

The null hypothesis states that no difference exists between prospective- and retrospective-rate determination for the cost variables. In other words, the states grouped according to prospective and retrospective reimbursement are not really separate populations but only subgroups of the same population. The results for skilled care are presented first, followed by the results for intermediate care.

Skilled Care.

Average Per Diem Cost. In all three years examined, the average per diem cost for skilled care is higher in those states using the retrospective method than in states using the prospective method (see table 4-7). In two of the three years the differences are statistically significant. In those two years the null hypothesis can be rejected, which means that prospective- and retrospective-rate setting did affect price. States that used prospective reimburse-

Table 4-7
Average Per Diem Cost (Prospective and Retrospective) for Medicaid—
Skilled Care

Year	Prospective	Retrospective	Level of Significance
1977	$23.69	$28.64	0.07
1976	22.38	25.74	0.21
1975	16.79	19.82	0.05

ment to calculate their payments for skilled care had significantly lower average per diem costs than did states that used the retrospective method. If it can be assumed that the quality of care delivered to patients is the same for both groups, then prospective reimbursement encourages the more-efficient delivery of skilled care to Medicaid patients.

Average Per Diem-Dollar Cost Increases. For both the 1976-1977 and 1975-1976 time periods, state Medicaid programs using retrospective-rate determination incurred greater cost increases for skilled care than did states using prospective reimbursement (see table 4-8). The differences, however, in average dollar cost increases were not statistically significant. The null hypothesis cannot be rejected for either time period. The conclusion is that prospective- and retrospective-rate determination did not affect the amount of dollar cost increases for skilled care during 1975 through 1977.

Intermediate Care.

Average Per Diem Cost. For all three years the average per diem cost for intermediate care was higher in those states using retrospective-rate determination when compared to states using the prospective method (see table 4-9). In all three years the differences were statistically significant, allowing the null hypothesis to be rejected. Prospective- and retrospective-rate setting did have an impact on the cost of intermediate care delivered to Medicaid patients during 1975 to 1977. If the quality of care delivered under both methods of rate calculation is assumed equal, then prospective reimbursement encourages the more-efficient delivery of intermediate care than does the retrospective method. If the quality of care delivered is not assumed equal, then the conclusion is that state Medicaid programs using prospective reimbursement paid less for intermediate care than did states using the retrospective method.

Average Per Diem-Dollar Cost Increases. For both the 1976-1977 and 1975-1976 time periods, state Medicaid programs that used the retrospec-

Table 4-8
Average Per Diem-Dollar Cost Increases (Prospective and Retrospective) for Medicaid—Skilled Care

Year	Prospective	Retrospective	Level of Significance
1976–1977	$1.85	$3.00	0.13
1975–1976	3.45	3.64	0.87

Table 4-9
Average Per Diem Cost for Medicaid—Intermediate Care

Year	Prospective	Retrospective	Level of Significance
1977	$17.54	$21.89	0.01
1976	16.10	19.98	0.02
1975	12.91	14.49	0.07

Table 4-10
Average Per Diem-Dollar Cost Increases for Medicaid—Intermediate Care

Year	Prospective	Retrospective	Level of Significance
1976–1977	$1.47	$2.38	0.12
1975–1976	2.54	3.30	0.69

tive-rate-setting method incurred greater dollar increases for intermediate care than did those states that used the prospective method (see table 4-10). The differences, however, between these reimbursement methods for average dollar cost increases were not statistically significant. For this reason the null hypothesis cannot be rejected. It must be concluded that prospective- and retrospective-rate determination did not affect the size of the annual dollar cost increases during 1975 through 1977.

Cost Conclusions

To summarize the impact of prospective- and retrospective-rate setting on the cost indexes, the major conclusion is that significant differences exist in the average per diem cost paid by state Medicaid programs using the two different methods. For both skilled care and intermediate care, from 1975 to 1977, states that calculated reimbursement prospectively paid lower per diem costs on average than did states that calculated payments retrospectively. Prospective-rate setting appears to be a more-effective method than the retrospective method for minimizing expenditures on long-term care.

The other cost index developed for this study measures the size of annual dollar cost increases. During both the 1976–1977 and the 1975–1976 time periods, for both skilled care and intermediate care, states using the retrospective method incurred larger annual cost increases. In all cases, however, the differences were not statistically significant, and the null hypothesis can not be rejected. From a statistical perspective, there was no difference in the size of the dollar cost increases between prospective- and retrospective-rate determination.

Rate-Determination Conclusions

Critics of prospective reimbursement have stated that this method may negatively affect the utilization of nursing-home care by Medicaid patients. The hypothesized danger is that prospective-rate setting could discourage long-term-care facilities from accepting Medicaid patients. No statistical difference was evident between prospective and retrospective reimbursement for the average number of Medicaid patients per 1,000 elderly nor for the average number of Medicaid patient days per 1,000 elderly for both skilled care and intermediate care. Nursing homes did not accept fewer Medicaid patients in those states using prospective reimbursement than in states using retrospective reimbursement. Also, there was no statistical difference in the average length of stay of Medicaid patients between the two methods for calculating payments for either skilled care or intermediate care. The conclusion of this analysis is that prospective and retrospective reimbursements do not affect the access of Medicaid patients to nursing-home care nor do these methods affect the length of stay.

The method of calculating payments does, however, have an impact on the average per diem cost of both skilled and intermediate care to state Medicaid programs. In all three years analyzed, the states' Medicaid programs that used the prospective-rate method paid a lower per diem cost for both skilled and intermediate care than did states using the retrospective method. In all but one year for skilled care, the cost differences between the two rate-setting methods were statistically significant. The major cost conclusion of this analysis is that states using prospective reimbursement paid a lower per diem cost for skilled care and intermediate care than did states using the retrospective method. Prospective-rate setting appears to be the better method for keeping down Medicaid expenditures on nursing-home care. In an analysis of cost increases, states using the retrospective method always had a larger dollar cost increase for both skilled and intermediate care. These differences, however, were never statistically significant.

Based on the analysis of cost data for 1975 to 1977, prospective-rate determination reimbursed nursing-home care at a significantly lower cost than did the retrospective method. At the same time, this analysis revealed that prospective reimbursement did not adversely affect Medicaid patients' access to long-term care.

Analysis of Reimbursement Methods

Do the different reimbursement methods have an impact on the cost and utilization indexes? What impact, if any, do reasonable-cost-related reimbursement, fixed-rate reimbursement, and negotiated-rate reimbursement have on the cost of care to state Medicaid patients for long-term care? (see appendix I for individual state listings for these cost and utilization indexes by reimbursement method.)

The analysis of utilization indexes for these reimbursement methods covers the period from 1973 to 1976. The data needed to develop the utilization indexes for 1977 and beyond were unavailable from the Department of Health and Human Services at the time of this study. The analysis of cost indexes is for the years 1973 to 1977.

Utilization Indexes

Does a statistically significant difference exist among reimbursement methods for the average number of Medicaid patients, 65 years and over, receiving skilled care per 1,000 of each state's elderly population? This analysis is an attempt to determine whether the different reimbursement methods affect Medicaid patients' access to skilled care. The null hypothesis declares that the states grouped according to the reasonable-cost, fixed-rate, and negotiated-rate methods are not really separate populations but subgroups of the same population. In other words, the null hypothesis proposes that no statistically significant differences exist in the averages for the different utilization indexes among states using the three different reimbursement methods. The impact of the reimbursement methods on the utilization measures are presented first for skilled care and then for intermediate care.

Skilled Care.

Medicaid Patients. In all four years, 1973–1976, the differences in the average number of Medicaid patients receiving skilled care per 1,000 elderly
among the different reimbursement methods are statistically significant,
allowing the null hypothesis to be rejected (see table 4–11). For skilled care
the type of reimbursement method does affect the average number of
Medicaid patients receiving skilled care per 1,000 elderly. What is particularly striking is the low average number of Medicaid patients per 1,000
elderly receiving skilled care in states using the negotiated-rate method for
Medicaid reimbursement. The entire trend for the negotiated-rate method is
also significant. In states using this method to pay for skilled care, the
number of Medicaid patients per 1,000 elderly has steadily declined since
1973 from 13.4 per 1,000 to 3.0 during 1976. This utilization index demonstrates that in those states that paid for skilled care with the negotiated-rate
method, fewer Medicaid patients are receiving skilled care in each successive
year. This information raises the question: Are Medicaid patients receiving
the necessary level of care in those states using the negotiated-rate method?
Are Medicaid patients denied proper care because of reimbursement practices?

Medicaid Patient Days. In two of the four years, 1974 and 1976, the differences in group means for the average number of Medicaid patients days of
skilled care per 1,000 elderly among the different reimbursement methods
are statistically significant, allowing the null hypothesis to be rejected (see
table 4–12). This means that the type of reimbursement method did affect
this consumption measure for skilled care during 1974 and 1976. Again,
what is striking is the low average number of Medicaid patient days per
1,000 population in states reimbursing skilled care with the negotiated-rate
method. The trend also reveals a pronounced drop in this utilization
measure from 1973 to 1976 in states using the negotiated-rate method. This
again raises the question: Did Medicaid patients in states using negotiated-
rate reimbursement receive the proper level of care?

Average Length of Stay. The type of reimbursement method did not affect
the average length of stay of Medicaid patients receiving skilled care (see
table 4–13). These observed outcomes could have occurred by chance 90 out
of every 100 times in 1973, 38 out of every 100 times in 1974, 99 out of every
100 times in 1975, and 67 out of every 100 times in 1976.

Intermediate Care.

Medicaid Patients. In only one year, 1973, did a statistically significant
difference exist among reimbursement methods for the average number of

Table 4–11
Medicaid Patients (Aged 65 and over) per 1,000 Elderly —
Skilled Care

Method	1976	1975	1974	1973
Reasonable-Cost related	16.8	17.6	16.1	12.5
Fixed rate	22.6	22.9	27.4	25.9
Negotiated rate	3.0	3.7	8.5	13.4
Average	16.6	17.3	18.7	16.1
Level of significance	0.05	0.07	0.03	0.06

Table 4–12
Medicaid Patient Days (Aged 65 and over) per 1,000 Elderly —
Skilled Care

Method	1976	1975	1974	1973
Reasonable-cost related	3,167	3,547	3,296	2,650
Fixed rate	4,238	3,896	5,548	5,280
Negotiated rate	518	652	956	2,897
Average	3,116	3,316	3,633	3,554
Level of significance	0.08	0.15	0.02	0.12

Table 4–13
Average Length of Stay for Medicaid Patients (Aged 65 and over)—
Skilled Care

Method	1976	1975	1974	1973
Reasonable-cost related	161	168	177	163
Fixed rate	170	169	194	176
Negotiated rate	140	165	138	174
Average	161	168	177	168
Level of significance	0.67	0.99	0.38	0.90

Medicaid patients receiving intermediate care per 1,000 elderly (see table 4-14). Unlike skilled care, the reimbursement method does not appear to affect the average number of Medicaid patients receiving intermediate care per 1,000 elderly. What is interesting to note, however, is that the average for this utilization index in states using the negotiated-rate method to reimburse for intermediate care was always the highest in all years. This is just the reverse for the skilled-care findings, when the average for states using the negotiated-rate method was always the lowest. States using the negotiated-rate method of reimbursement for nursing-home care had fewer Medicaid patients per 1,000 elderly receiving skilled care and more Medicaid patients per 1,000 receiving intermediate care than with the other two reimbursement methods.

Medicaid Patient Days. In only one year, 1974, did a statistically significant difference exist among reimbursement methods for the average number of Medicaid patient days of intermediate care per 1,000 elderly (see table 4-15). Unlike skilled care, the reimbursement method does not appear to affect the average number of Medicaid patient days per 1,000 elderly for intermediate care. Again, however, it is interesting to note that the average for this index in states using the negotiated-rate method for intermediate care was always the highest for all reimbursement methods.

Average Length of Stay. In all but one year, 1973, no statistically significant difference existed in the average length of stay for Medicaid patients receiving intermediate care among the different reimbursement methods. Given this one exception, the reimbursement method does not appear to affect average length of stay for intermediate-care Medicaid patients.

Utilization Conclusions

The type of reimbursement method did have a pronounced impact on the average number of Medicaid patients receiving skilled care per 1,000 elderly. In states that reimbursed with the negotiated-rate method, the average number of Medicaid patients in skilled-care facilities per 1,000 elderly declined from 13.4 patients per 1,000 elderly in 1973 to 3.0 patients per 1,000 elderly in 1976. In states using the negotiated-rate method, the average number of Medicaid patient days of skilled care per 1,000 elderly declined from 2,897 patient days per 1,000 elderly in 1973 to 518 patient days per 1,000 elderly in 1976. These ratios demonstrate a dramatic drop in the utilization of skilled care by Medicaid patients in states that used the negotiated-rate method of reimbursement. States using the negotiated-rate method to reimburse intermediate-care facilities always had the highest

Table 4–14
Medicaid Patients (Aged 65 and over) per 1,000 Elderly —
Intermediate Care

Method	1976	1975	1974	1973
Reasonable-cost related	25.2	22.0	21.9	20.5
Fixed rate	25.7	23.3	20.6	18.9
Negotiated rate	32.2	36.2	34.3	41.3
Average	26.1	23.9	22.8	22.7
Level of significance	0.58	0.14	0.15	0.14

Table 4–15
Medicaid Patient Days (Aged 65 and over) per 1,000 Elderly —
Intermediate Care

Method	1976	1975	1974	1973
Reasonable-cost related	5,819	5,256	5,159	4,261
Fixed rate	6,486	6,158	4,660	3,581
Negotiated rate	8,145	7,666	8,854	8,841
Average	6,293	5,760	5,396	4,399
Level of significance	0.54	0.43	0.10	0.21

Table 4–16
Average Length of Stay for Medicaid Patients (Aged 65 and over)—
Intermediate Care

Method	1976	1975	1974	1973
Reasonable-cost related	234	230	229	237
Fixed rate	226	236	209	143
Negotiated rate	241	212	242	219
Average	233	229	224	197
Level of significance	0.82	0.60	0.38	0.01

average numbers of Medicaid patients receiving intermediate care per 1,000 elderly and the highest average numbers of Medicaid patient days of intermediate care per 1,000 elderly than the other reimbursement methods from 1973 through 1976.

The major conclusion concerning the impact the different reimbursement methods have had on the utilization of long-term care is that states using the negotiated-rate method consistently had fewer Medicaid patients receiving skilled care and more Medicaid patients receiving intermediate care when compared to states using the other payment methods. This conclusion suggests that in states using the negotiated-rate method, patients who in other states would have received skilled care were actually placed in intermediate-care facilities. These data raise an important question: Are Medicaid patients denied access to needed skilled care and improperly placed in intermediate-care facilities in states using negotiated-rate reimbursement? Or, in states using the other reimbursement methods, is skilled care overconsumed by Medicaid patients? In other words, are some Medicaid patients improperly placed in skilled-care facilities when intermediate care is really all they need? An analysis of per diem–reimbursement rates for skilled care and intermediate care, by type of reimbursement method, should help answer these questions.

Cost Indexes

Does a significant difference exist in the average per diem price paid for long-term care among states using the different reimbursement methods? The null hypothesis states that no difference exists in the average per diem costs among the three different reimbursement methods. In other words, the states grouped according to the three different reimbursement methods are not really separate populations but actually subgroups of the same population. For this reason the null hypothesis assumes that average per diem costs do not differ significantly among reimbursement methods. The results for skilled care are presented first, followed by the results for intermediate care.

Skilled Care.

Average Per Diem Cost. After looking at table 4–17, one thing becomes obvious: Every year the per diem price of skilled care increased for all reimbursement methods. The average per diem price for skilled care was always the highest in states that used the reasonable-cost-related method and always lowest in states that used the negotiated-rate method. In statistical terms during 1973, 1975, and 1976 the differences in average per diem costs among the three different reimbursement methods were significant. In 1974

Table 4–17
Average Per Diem Cost for Medicaid—Skilled Care

Method	1977	1976	1975	1974	1973
Reasonable-cost related	$26.05	$24.78	$19.87	$15.19	$14.52
Fixed rate	20.22	19.00	16.80	13.70	13.39
Negotiated rate	15.33	15.03	12.37	9.80	9.42
Average	24.80	22.97	18.68	14.25	13.62
Level of significance	0.11	0.05	0.06	0.11	0.08

Table 4–18
Average Per Diem–Dollar Cost Increases for Medicaid—Skilled Care

Method	1976–1977	1975–1976	1974–1975	1973–1974
Reasonable-cost related	$2.63	$3.51	$4.92	$0.69
Fixed rate	1.07	2.21	2.68	0.73
Negotiated rate	0.08	2.66	2.57	0.41
Average	2.30	3.20	4.22	0.68
Level of significance	0.18	0.37	0.20	0.87

and 1977 the differences among groups were just barely above the stated level of significance. Given the consistency in trend and the magnitude of the observed per diem–cost outcomes, this analysis concludes that for skilled care the type of reimbursement method used does affect the level of payment. The reasonable-cost-related method is consistently associated with the highest level of payment, and the negotiated-rate method is consistently associated with the lowest level of payment.

Average Per Diem–Dollar Cost Increases. During none of the cost-change time periods was the difference in the average dollar cost increases among reimbursement methods statistically significant (see table 4–18). Reimbursement has no statistical impact on the size of cost increases for skilled care based on the data analyzed in this study. One interesting generalization drawn from these observed outcomes is that in all time periods, except 1973-1974, the reasonable-cost-related method had the largest annual dollar cost increases, although none was statistically significant.

Intermediate Care.

Average Per Diem Cost. For the years 1973 through 1976 no statistical differences existed among reimbursement methods for the average per diem cost of intermediate care (see table 4–19). In 1977 a statistically significant difference did exist among reimbursement methods. The results for 1977, however, may be biased by the fact that only two states used the negotiated-rate method to reimburse intermediate-care facilities. The average per diem cost for intermediate care in Hawaii was $39.05 during 1977, and the average per diem cost for this level of care in Oklahoma was $13.99, yielding an average for the negotiated-rate method of $26.52 for 1977. The major conclusion of this analysis is that no significant differences were evident in average per diem costs for intermediate care among reimbursement methods.

Average Per Diem–Dollar Cost Increases. In all time periods, except 1974–1975, the differences among reimbursement methods for average per diem-dollar cost increases for intermediate care were not statistically significant (see table 4–40). The reimbursement method usually had no impact on the magnitude of cost increases for intermediate care. No generalizations can be made about which reimbursement method consistently had the largest average dollar cost increase because this leadership role shifted among reimbursement methods. These data reinforce the conclusion that reimbursement method has no impact on the size of average dollar cost increases for intermediate care.

Cost Conclusion

Statistically significant differences existed in average per diem costs for skilled care among reimbursement methods. The major cost conclusion is that the different methods of payment did have an impact on the average per diem costs paid by state Medicaid programs to skilled-care facilities. The different reimbursement methods did not have an impact on the average dollar cost increase for either skilled or intermediate care. The different reimbursement methods did not affect the average per diem cost paid by state Medicaid programs to intermediate-care facilities.

Summary

The type of reimbursement method had a significant impact on the average number of Medicaid patients receiving skilled care per 1,000 elderly. In those states that reimbursed skilled care with the negotiated-rate method, the average number of Medicaid patients per 1,000 receiving skilled care

Table 4-19
Average Per Diem Cost for Medicaid—Intermediate Care

Method	1977	1976	1975	1974	1973
Reasonable-cost related	$17.94	$17.09	$14.56	$10.04	$8.98
Fixed rate	17.55	16.47	13.20	10.08	8.50
Negotiated rate	26.52	16.21	12.42	10.50	8.13
Average	18.24	16.83	14.00	10.11	8.69
Level of significance	0.05	0.92	0.39	0.98	0.86

Table 4-20
Average Per Diem-Dollar Cost Increases for Medicaid—Intermediate Care

Method	1976-1977	1975-1976	1974-1975	1973-1974
Reasonable-cost related	$1.71	$2.31	$4.54	$1.06
Fixed rate	1.48	3.28	2.44	1.42
Negotiated rate	2.88	3.79	2.31	0.70
Average	1.72	2.73	3.68	1.17
Level of significance	0.55	0.51	0.04	0.88

was markedly lower than in the other states that used different reimbursement methods. Although not statistically significant, the average number of Medicaid patients receiving intermediate care was consistently greater in states using the negotiated-rate method of reimbursement than in states using other methods. These data suggest that Medicaid patients, who in other states would have received skilled care, were placed in intermediate-care facilities in states using the negotiated-rate method. Was skilled care overutilized in states using the reasonable-cost-related and fixed-rate methods of reimbursement? Or, are some Medicaid patients denied access to needed skilled care and placed in intermediate-care facilities in states using negotiated-rate reimbursement?

This chapter suggested earlier that the analysis of per diem–payment rates by type of reimbursement may help answer these questions. Significant differences existed among reimbursement methods for average per diem rates paid for skilled care. In all years, states using the negotiated-rate method consistently had the lowest average per diem payment for skilled care. Conversely, there were no statistically significant differences among reimbursement methods for the average per diem rate paid by Medicaid to intermediate-care facilities.

These data lead to the conclusion that in states using the negotiated-rate method, the inadequacy of per diem payments for skilled care has caused skilled-care facilities to refuse to accept Medicaid patients. The annually decreasing number of Medicaid patients receiving skilled care in these states supports this conclusion. Beverly Enterprises, a large, proprietary long-term-care chain, plans to limit the number of Medicaid patients it accepts in order to increase the number of private patients it services to increase per-patient revenues.[5] The Four Seasons Nursing Homes division of the Anta Corporation has announced to its shareholders that it is increasing the percentage of private patients in its nursing centers, which is another indication of the current reluctance of the industry to accept Medicaid patients.[6]

A final indication that the low payment rates in states using the negotiated-rate method have locked Medicaid patients out of skilled-care facilities is a 1975 study of the nursing-home system in Virginia.[7] This study noted a drop in the number of skilled-care beds participating in the Virginia Medicaid program from 1,525 beds in 34 facilities during 1973 to 1,309 beds in 27 facilities during 1974. The conclusion drawn was that the 5.95-percentage increase in per diem rates for skilled care was insufficient to keep these beds participating in the Medicaid program. Interestingly, the number of intermediate-care beds increased from 6,577 beds in 88 facilities during 1973 to 8,922 beds in 110 facilities during 1974, following a more-generous 13.3-percentage increase between years in the per diem rate for intermediate care (see table 4-21).

Table 4-21
Long-Term-Care Facilities Reimbursed by Medicaid in Virginia

Type of Facility	1973	1974	Percent of Increase (Decrease)
Skilled nursing care			
Number of facilities	34	27	(21)
Number of beds	1525	1309	(14)
Average per diem– patient cost	$25.53	$27.05	5.95
Ceiling per diem cost	$38.30	$40.58	5.95
Intermediate care			
Number of facilities	88	110	25
Number of beds	6577	8922	38.6
Average per diem– patient cost	$17.10	$19.37	13.3
Ceiling per diem cost	$25.65	$29.05	13.3

Source: Virginia State Health Department, "Nursing Home Cost Comparisons," January 1975 computations for Medicaid reimbursement.

Nationally, no statistically significant differences were evident among reimbursement methods for the average per diem rate paid by the state Medicaid programs to intermediate-care facilities. These data support the conclusion that the Medicaid patients in negotiated-rate states, who were denied access to skilled care, were placed in intermediate-care facilities. This analysis demonstrates that inadequate Medicaid-payment rates can affect the utilization of long-term care by Medicaid patients.

Notes

1. Hubert Blalock, *Social Statistics* (New York: McGraw-Hill, 1960); Gudmund Iverson and Helmut Norpoth, *Analysis of Variance* (Beverly Hills: Sage Publications, 1976); Jack Levin, *Elementary Statistics in Social Research* (New York: Harper and Row, 1973); and John Phillips, *Statistical Thinking* (San Francisco: W.H. Freeman, 1973).

2. Levin, *Elementary Statistics,* p. 142.

3. Sanford Labovitz, "Criteria for Selecting a Significance Level: A Note on the Sacredness of .05," *The American Sociologist* 3-4 (August 1968):221.

4. Applied Management Sciences, *Report on Systems of Reimbursement for Long-Term Care: vol. I: Analysis and Recommendations,* 7 April 1976, pp. 2.1-2.9.

5. "Nursing the Nursing Homes Back to Health," *Business Week,* 5 December 1977, p. 70.

6. Anta Corporation, "Third Quarter Report for the Nine Months Ended March 31, 1979," Oklahoma City, Oklahoma.

7. Robert J. Buchanan, "Public Policy and Long-Term Care," (Master's thesis, University of Virginia, May 1976), appendix II-A, p. 122.

5 PL 92–603 (Section 249)

The Medicaid system, administered by a collection of semiautonomous state programs, had spawned by 1972 a variety of reimbursement methods and a wide range of payment rates for nursing-home care. Prior to 1972 one thread common to most Medicaid programs was dissatisfaction with the reimbursement system. The long-term-care industry was concerned with what it claimed were inadequate Medicaid payments. Consumer groups and government officials were concerned that the reimbursement methods used by some state programs did not promote the efficient delivery of high-quality health care. Many state-government administrators were concerned with the rising costs of long-term care to their Medicaid programs.

In 1972 Congress enacted PL 92–603 that amended the Social Security Act. Section 249 of the new law amended Title XIX of the Social Security Act to require all state Medicaid programs to reimburse long-term-care facilities on a "reasonable-cost-related basis" effective 1 July 1976. What caused Section 249 to be enacted? How was dissatisfaction with the previous reimbursement system channeled into the political process? What groups were the principal actors in the policy process, and how did they articulate their preferences for change?

Policy-Process Model

A policymaking model serves as a useful framework to describe what actions precipitate change in public policy. First, as an overview of the public-policy process, Ripley, Moreland, and Sennereich have developed a systems model labeled the "government-policy arena."[1] The government-policy arena contains three basic elements: (1) structure, (2) environment, and (3) policy response. Structure consists of all the "characteristics, norms, and recurring patterns" inside the government. This concept of structure is also known as "the black box." Environment is everything outside the boundaries of the governmental structure. Policy response is the output resulting from the government's reactions to the environment and the workings of its own structures. According to this model, the policy process works when feedback and inputs, generated from the environment, are channeled into the structures of government. The structures process these inputs and create public policy in response.

The subgovernment model adds another dimension to the description of policy formulation.[2] Subgovernments are "clusters of individuals that effectively make most of the routine decisions in a given substantive area of policy."[3] At the national level, the clusters of individuals that populate the subgovernments are members of the U.S. House of Representatives and the Senate, members of congressional staffs, members of the executive branch connected with the issue, and private-interest groups with an interest in the policy output.

Synthesizing the political-systems model and the subgovernment model, public policy is formulated in separate policy arenas or subgovernments. Each policy arena/subgovernment works with relatively separate sets of substantive issues. Affected groups and individuals interject inputs and feedback into these policy arenas, expressing their preferences for public-policy outputs that will benefit their interests. The appropriate subgovernment processes these inputs and formulates public policy. The resulting public policy is the product of the interaction among subcommittees of Congress and their staffs, the bureaus of the executive branch, and interest groups from the environment.

Relating these models to Section 249 of PL 92–603, what conditions in the environment caused which political actors to make demands on the structures of government for policy changes? Which institutions of what subgovernment interact to create the policy output? This policy-arena/subgovernment model provides an analytical framework to describe the development of the amendment to the Social Security Act that required all state Medicaid programs to reimburse nursing homes on a reasonable-cost-related basis.

Section 249 and the Policy Model

Section 249 was first introduced into the formal policy process at the Senate Finance Committee. According to that committee's report on the Social Security Act amendments of 1972, the committee was concerned "that some skilled-nursing facilities and ICFs are being overpaid by Medicaid, while others are being paid too little to support the quality of care that Medicaid patients are expected to need and receive."[4] The initial policy response proposed by the Senate Finance Committee was to have all state Medicaid programs reimburse long-term-care facilities on a reasonable-cost-related basis by 1 July 1974.

If nursing homes are underpaid, either because a rate of reimbursement is set unrealistically low or because the state program does not recognize as allowable costs all the true costs of care, then the institution would be under pressure to reduce the quantity and the quality of the services delivered. The

Senate Finance Committee was concerned that, at worst, nursing homes might refuse to accept Medicaid patients.[5]

Costs are not the same everywhere, and the committee was also concerned that a flat-rate method of reimbursement might set payment rates too high in some states or that a state program might recognize unnecessary items as allowable costs, thus providing little incentive for efficiency to the producers of long-term care. These inefficiencies and diseconomies in reimbursement by some state programs result in the waste of Medicaid resources. The Senate committee members feared that rising Medicaid costs, compounded by inefficiency in some reimbursement methods for nursing-home care, would cause some states to cut back on essential Medicaid-covered services or even drop out of the Medicaid program altogether.[6]

In terms of the policy-arena/subgovernment model, the Senate Finance Committee perceived problems with Medicaid reimbursement for long-term care based on feedback from the environment. According to Senator Carl Curtis of Nebraska, the ranking Republican on the Senate Finance Committee in 1978, "the recommendation for reasonable-cost reimbursement first appeared formally in a staff recommendation on 13 March 1972. . . . The majority staff was responsible for the proposal. . . ."[7]

According to a committee staff member, Section 249 was an internal, committee-generated idea. It was formulated because the Finance Committee and its staff "recognized the problems relating to the overpayment and underpayment for nursing-home care." Senator Curtis added another dimension to the reasons for the development of Section 249: The majority staff's "thesis was that reimbursement formulas for nursing homes should be on a similar footing to that of hospitals, which had been placed on a reasonable-cost-reimbursement formula under a similar recommendation." Jay Constantine, head of the health-professional staff for the Finance Committee, reinforced this perspective: "Probably the direct ancestor of Section 249 was the requirement in Medicare and Medicaid that hospitals be paid on a reasonable-cost basis. Another parent was the requirement that extended-care facilities be paid on a reasonable-cost basis under Medicare."[8]

The nursing-home industry had lobbied for a more-rational reimbursement system, but it did not directly initiate specific demand for the reasonable-cost-related policy in 1972. The American Nursing Home Association [presently called the American Health Care Association (AHCA)] "supported the inclusion of Section 249 in the 1972 amendments, mainly because it was deemed essential to have some kind of federal mandate which would discourage states from setting rates on a purely arbitrary basis. Of particular concern was the propensity of many states to ignore the effects of increases in the federal minimum wage and costly changes in health and safety standards for nursing homes being required by federal and state regulations."[9] The AHCA is an organization representing nursing homes, approximately 80 percent of them proprietary facilities.

The American Association of Homes for the Aging (AAHA), a national organization of nonprofit nursing homes, also testified for the reasonable-cost-related system in 1972. This organization had also been "active throughout the period of 1972 through 1976 to speed the implementation" of Section 249.[10]

In regard to nursing-home-industry input on Section 249 during Finance Committee deliberations, Senator Curtis stated, "Although some differed if they felt their current reimbursement formula was more favorable, trade associations were generally supportive of the proposal." Senator Curtis also commented, "At the time the [Nixon] administration was concerned about the proposal on a question of cost; I believe they did not formally take a position but expressed the need for greater flexibility [for state Medicaid programs]. I am advised they prevailed for a two-year delay (from July 1974 to July 1976) on implementation of the proposal." Interviews with individuals within the Medicaid Bureau support the statement by Senator Curtis that the DHHS did not take a formal position on Section 249. As individuals, however, many people within the bureau were concerned that Section 249 would increase Medicaid expenditures for long-term care.

Based on interviews with Senator Curtis, staff members for the Senate Finance Committee, long-term-care trade-association spokespeople, and Medicaid Bureau officials, this study concludes that the formal proposal for reasonable-cost reimbursement for long-term care resulted from the efforts of the majority staff of the Senate Finance Committee. The motivation was to make Medicaid reimbursement for nursing-home care consistent with Medicare and Medicaid reasonable-cost reimbursement for hospital care.

Laurence Lane, the director for Public Policy at the AAHA, stated that considerable informal interaction occcurred between congressional committees and trade associations in the development of the legislative ancestors of Section 249. This suggests that the long-term-care industry had an important indirect role in the development of Section 249.

Senator Moss first introduced the idea of reasonable-cost reimbursement during 1967 as an amendment to the Social Security Act. According to Laurence Lane, the senator "got the idea for a cost-related amendment from a former staffer on the Senate Special Committee on Aging. . . . [The staffer] worked on the Aging Committee during the early sixties when it performed the complete study of the Kerr-Mills program as a forerunner and important resource document to the Medicare and Medicaid programs."

According to the director for Public Policy at the AAHA, the AAHA "was deeply involved, through the interaction of several of its key members, with the staffers. . . . There were informal linkages which extended beyond the formal ones such as testifying and letter writing which indicate a collaborative effort. The zeal for the cost-related posture was influenced by the New York State operationalizing of a cost-related system under the Kerr-Mills program. [The trade association] had a strong base in New York and was closely linked with key state officials who were informally linked to the Senate staffers.''

Reasonable-cost reimbursement for hospitals by Medicare and Medicaid was the legislative ancestor of Section 249. Through formal and informal linkages with congressional staffers, at least one trade association actively worked and pushed for the development of these legislative ancestors. Although trade associations may not have directly initiated the demand for Section 249, at least one long-term-care association, the AAHA, actually helped formulate reasonable-cost reimbursement for Medicare and Medicaid payments for hospital care. The zeal for reasonable-cost reimbursement was based upon the association's favorable experience with this type of reimbursement in New York State under the Kerr-Mills program.

Informal relationships between trade associations and congressional staff have been important in the development of Medicare and Medicaid reimbursement policies. These informal friendships and relationships indicate "the collaborative development of programs." There is a flow of people from government positions to trade associations. The AAHA representative developed his legislative experience, skills, and contacts while he was a staff member in Congress before working for the nursing-home industry. The Senate staffer who introduced Senator Moss to reasonable-cost reimbursement is presently a private long-term-care consultant. An important source of information for this research within the Health Care Finance Administration, the parent organization of the Medicare and Medicaid Bureaus, is presently working for a health-care trade association. Their expertise in both the formal and informal workings of policy formulation and administration, developed while working for government, helps explain the importance of the informal networks of "friendship groupings which indicate collaborative developments of programs," as the director for Public Policy at the AAHA stated.

No equivalent of Section 249 was in the House version of the 1972 Social Security amendments. The House/Senate Conference Committee, due to concern for the ability of state programs to comply with deadlines, reported out a bill that delayed implementation of the Senate-passed proposal until 1 July 1976.[11] When passed by both houses of Congress and signed by President Nixon, 1 July 1976 became the implementation date mandated by federal law.

In September 1977, Senator Bellmon of Oklahoma declared, in a statement read into *The Congressional Record,* that many state Medicaid programs were having problems preparing and submitting reimbursement plans for approval by the DHHS as required by statute. By autumn 1977 only two state plans had been approved. The remaining states either had not submitted plans, had to modify their plans, or had their plans under review.[12]

Implementation was effectively delayed until 1 January 1978 by the secretary of DHHS. Dr. Paul Willging, the acting director of the Medicaid Bureau, explained the department's reasons for the delay beyond the statutory date. First, "the department's regulations implementing the statutory requirements were not published in final form until 1 July 1976, the effective date."[13] The state Medicaid programs were required to develop their reasonable-cost-related-reimbursement plans for long-term care based on these department regulations. "1 January 1978 was the date set in the regulations by which the states were to establish reasonable-cost-related rates, on the basis of cost data submitted by providers. The interim period was necessary to allow for the accumulation of cost data [by the Medicaid programs on nursing-home operations in their states]." According to Dr. Willging, by December 1978 only three states had not yet had their plans approved.

The Medicaid director also stated that "the timetable set forth in the [DHHS] regulations did not delay the effective date of the statute, but merely committed the department, for a limited time, not to impose a sanction. . . . Nothing in the regulations discouraged the states from implementing the statute immediately, and indeed the preamble to the regulations encouraged the states to do so." However, the fact that the department's final regulations, developed to guide state programs in developing reasonable-cost reimbursement, were not published until 1 July 1976, made it difficult for the state programs to obtain department approval for their plans by the 1 July 1976 statutory deadline. As is discussed later in this chapter, the authority of the secretary to delay implementation has been challenged by the long-term-care associations in the federal courts.

The Bellmon Amendment

In September 1977 Senator Bellmon of Oklahoma introduced on the Senate floor an amendment to HR 3, the Medicare and Medicaid Antifraud and Abuse bill. The amendment had two objectives."[14] First, it was intended to delay implementation of Section 249 until 1 January 1978 because of state compliance difficulties. Second, the amendment was intended to relieve state Medicaid programs from any retroactive liability for reasonable-cost-related reimbursement back to 1 July 1976, the original implementation date of Section 249. HR 3, with the Bellmon amendment, was passed by the U.S. Senate.

The National Council of State Public Welfare Administrators (NCSPWA) of the American Public Welfare Association (APWA) supported the Bellmon amendment.[15] The NCSPWA is an association of administrators from all state welfare agencies, who have the primary administrative responsibility for the Medicaid program. This group supported the Bellmon amendment because it gave the states additional time to comply with federal regulations, and it would absolve the state Medicaid programs of possible fiscal liability for DHHS's delay in implementing Section 249.

Associations representing long-term-care facilities were strongly opposed to any implementation delay. The exception was a group from the senator's home state, the Oklahoma State Nursing Home Association. This association did not want to change that state's negotiated-rate method of Medicaid reimbursement for long-term care. Through parliamentary maneuver, and a sooner-than-expected vote on HR 3 due to a break in the energy-bill filibuster, the Senate approved the delay in implementing Section 249 until 1 January 1978. The industry groups had been caught off guard by the swiftness of the Senate action.

Since the House version of HR 3 contained no equivalent of the Bellmon amendment, the AAHA, the National Council of Health Care Services, and the AHCA lobbied intensively with the House/Senate Conference Committee to delete the Bellmon amendment. The AAHA, which represents nonprofit nursing homes, argued that delay in implementation would reward bureaucratic inertia and discourage efforts to improve the quality of nursing-home care.[16] The associations were successful in removing the Bellmon amendment from the Medicare and Medicaid Antifraud and Abuse bill. Thus, in the fall of 1977, organizations representing long-term-care institutions defeated an attempt, by statute, to delay the implementation date of Section 249 from 1 July 1976 to 1 January 1978.

Most of the state Medicaid programs, however, were still not in compliance with the law late in 1977, over one year beyond the date mandated by law. As is discussed later in this chapter, Section 249 and the implementation delay has created considerable legal activity against both the DHHS and various state Medicaid programs.

Group Theory and the Policy Model

The group-theory model of policymaking, applied to the policy-arena/subgovernment framework, gives insight into the study of the Bellmon amendment in the policy process. The basic premise of group theory is that interaction among groups "is the central fact of politics."[17] The policy-arena/subgovernment model adds that policy is made in separate substantive arenas. Interest groups interject inputs into these subgovernments to influence policy outcomes. In the case of the Bellmon amendment, the APWA, representing Medicaid administrators, supported the implementation delay of Section 249. Also, the Oklahoma State Nursing Home Association, which preferred Oklahoma's negotiated-rate payment system to Section 249's reasonable-cost-related method, supported the amendment introduced by Senator Bellmon. The major representatives of the nursing-home industry actively lobbied to kill the Bellmon amendment in the conference committee.

The group-theory model of politics views the official policymakers— the men and women operating the institutions of government—as responding to inputs from competing groups. The black box, or structures of government, processes the conflicting inputs and creates policy. According to group theory, public policy at a given point in time is a balance of equilibrium of the influence and power of interested groups.[18] In the struggle over the Bellmon amendment, opponents of delay were able to channel sufficient inputs into the policy arena/subgovernment to defeat the amendment.

One final point on the policymaking process in the United States: PL 92–603 is a good illustration of how the policymaking process has fragmented into separate policy arenas or subgovernments. PL 92–603 is a complex law containing 413 sections.[19] The provisions of the law range from old-age insurance to health-related Medicare and Medicaid issues. This is just one of many laws the Ninety-Second Congress and the president considered in 1972. To develop the expertise to make effective policy, policymakers must specialize. The executive branch of government is organized according to substantive specialty. The Congress specializes through the committee and subcommittee system, also organized along substantive lines. This need for specialization in order to develop expertise is what creates the separate policy arenas or subgovernments of the U.S. policy-making process.

Implementation of Section 249

PL 92–603 (Section 249) amended the Social Security Act to include the following passage:

> [E]ffective 1 July 1976, for payment of the skilled-nursing-facility and intermediate-care-facility services provided under the plan [Medicaid] on a reasonable-cost-related basis, as determined in accordance with the methods and standards which shall be developed by the state on the basis of cost-finding methods as approved and verified by the secretary . . .[20]

To implement Section 249 each state participating in the Medicaid program must submit to the DHHS a state plan outlining its proposed payment principles. The states can either adopt the reimbursement methods used by the Medicare program or they can develop their own methods.[21] If a state plan adopts the Medicare principles of reimbursement, then DHHS will grant automatic approval. This is not an attractive option to many state programs, however, because according to Dr. Willging, the director of the Medicaid program, many states view the Medicare definition of reasonable cost as inflationary.[22] All other reasonable-cost-related-payment methods must be approved by the regional commissioner or the DHHS's Social and Rehabilitation Service. The delay of the states in submitting these plans for approval caused the secretary of DHHS to postpone implementation of Section 249 from 1 July 1976 until 1 January 1978.

DHHS Guidelines for State Plans

DHHS provided guidelines to the state Medicaid programs that chose to develop their own definition of the reasonable-cost-related method.[23] The guidelines are:

1. The plan must describe requirements for cost finding and cost reporting by the providers of long-term-care services.
2. The plan must provide for audits to verify the accuracy and reasonableness of cost reports furnished by these providers.
3. The plan must identify the items of expense which are allowable and reimbursable costs under the state program.
4. The plan must identify the methods and standards which will be used by the state program to determine reasonable-cost-related-reimbursement rates. The plan must begin payment on the basis of such methods and standards no later than 1 January 1978.
5. The plan must provide that the state will pay for long-term-care services in the amount determined by the methods and standards.

Legislative Intent and State Plans

The legislative history of Section 249 gives additional guidance to the state Medicaid programs in their development of state plans for nursing-home reimbursement. The Senate Finance Committee wanted the states to have flexibility in developing their own reasonable-cost-related method and not necessarily be restricted to Medicare reimbursement principles that can be "detailed," "expensive," and "cumbersome."[24] The Senate report on the Social Security amendments explicitly gives the state plans the freedom to set rates "on a geographic basis [by region within the state], a class basis [type of care delivered], or on an institution-by-institution basis." Finally, another important guide to the states is the implication in the Senate report that states are to be allowed to set rates prospectively without provision for retrospective adjustment.

To summarize the legislative intent of Section 249, the Senate Finance Committee wanted the states to have flexibility to define allowable costs and to set a value on these costs. The legislative history makes clear that the states are "to be free in setting their reasonable-cost-related payments to take into account, on the one hand, incentives toward efficiency, and on the other hand, incentives to upgrade the quality of care."[25]

Section 249 and Legal Action

The implementation of Section 249 has created considerable controversy, resulting in many legal battles. These suits have focused on two important implementation decisions made by the DHHS. One debate revolves around the question of profit in long-term-care reimbursement. The other relates to the secretary's delay from 1 July 1976 to 1 January 1978 in implementing Section 249.

AHCA, Inc. v. Califano

The suit brought by the AHCA against Secretary Califano in December 1977 "was essentially a challenge to the secretary's authority to severely restrict the right of states to permit nursing homes to realize a reasonable profit from providing care to medical-assistance recipients."[26]

The 1 July 1976 federal regulations for implementing Section 249 did not mention the profit issue. The accompanying preamble, however, explained how profits could be earned by nursing homes from the delivery of care to Medicaid recipients. Those facilities that had operating costs less than the rate they received as part of a class of facilities could keep the difference as a profit. Since only six state programs reimbursed nursing homes on a class basis at that time, "the opportunity to earn a profit under this policy would have been effectively foreclosed to nursing homes in other states."[27]

In addition, the preamble provided that a return on a "proprietary owner's net equity is the only item of profit that may be included as an allowable cost."[28] At issue here was whether nonprofit nursing homes could earn a return on equity. The AHCA claims that nonprofit institutions need this return on equity to expand the delivery of their services. In summary, the suit brought by the AHCA against Secretary Califano argued that the "secretary has illegally restricted the ability of states to include a profit or similar incentives in its payments to health-care institutions for services rendered."[29]

The secretary of DHHS argued that "the final regulations do contain a mechanism for profit compensation."[30] When a state establishes its reasonable-cost-related method for reimbursement, the secretary maintained, it could utilize a rate of reimbursement on a facility-by-facility basis or on a classwide basis. (Although not mentioned in the suit, the legislative history of 249 makes clear that states can also set rates on a geographical basis.)[31] Providers "who minimize expenses may realize a profit in the amount by which those expenses undercut the applicable rate."[32] The secretary went on to express his objection to the inclusion of profit as an allowable cost item. The secretary favored prospective-rate setting because he believed it established a better incentive for the efficient supply of services.

Judge Pratt, in his decision, dismissed the AHCA's suit against the secretary. The judge ruled that the "existing statutory and regulatory program does allow states to build a profit mechanism into the reimbursement scheme."[33] State flexibility in establishing reimbursement methods may not be as great as the AHCA desired, but Judge Pratt further concluded that this was the "overriding intent of Congress" in passing Section 249. The court ruled that the secretary had followed "statutory directive" in implementing Section 249. Therefore, the court could "not substitute its judgment or the plaintiff's judgment for that of the secretary in determining which method is preferable." Judge Pratt further concluded that the DHHS's regulatory method was "a reasonable one: it endorses a profit concept for efficient providers of services while establishing a ceiling upon total reimbursement."

In concluding his decision, Judge Pratt declared that the preamble of "basis and purpose" that accompanied the final regulations, did not provide sufficient guidance to enable state administrators to comply with the regulations concerning opportunities for profit. The court ordered the secretary to issue a statement of basis and purpose within sixty days that "shall serve to advise interested parties of the intended operation of the regulations" concerning profit.

This statement was published in the *Federal Register* on 6 February 1978. This clarification reaffirmed, as upheld by the federal district court, that a return on net equity can be treated as an allowable cost only for proprietary nursing homes. Return on net equity is "not an appropriate element in the calculation of reimbursement rates for nonprofit and government providers."[34] The state program is free to set the rate of return for profit institutions at the rate it "calculates is necessary to attract and maintain adequate investment in the nursing-home industry."

This statement further clarified that state plans may also use two other approaches, separately or in combination, to provide profit to nonprofit as well as to profit homes. These methods are class rates, or prospective rates, set either on a facility or class-of-care basis. Proprietary and nonproprietary nursing homes could earn a profit equal to the difference between the set rate and their actual cost.

Alabama Nursing Home Association v. Califano

The Alabama Nursing Home Association (ANHA) brought suit against DHHS Secretary Califano in the federal district court challenging the validity of the then-current method used by the Alabama Medicaid program to reimburse long-term-care facilities.[35] The ANHA argued in its challenge that the regulations for implementing reasonable-cost-related reimbursement were not in compliance with federal law, as stated in Section 249. The suit specifically challenged the secretary's decision to delay the implementation date of reasonable-cost-related reimbursement.

The federal district court ruled that DHHS was not authorized to change the implementation date of Section 249 from 1 July 1976 to 1 January 1978, declaring the latter date invalid. The court further ruled that the inability of the state program to pay for care under the new regulations did not excuse the state program from compliance with the law. The court found no provision, either explicit or implicit, in the Social Security Act that allowed a state to alter federal standards to satisfy a state's budgetary dilemma.[36] Since state participation in the Medicaid program is voluntary, the court reasoned, financial inability to meet federal regulations does not excuse a state from compliance.

Additional Legal Action

Additional suits were brought against either Secretary Califano or state officials by individual nursing homes or their associations in a number of states challenging the delay in implementing Section 249. On 8 October 1977 the federal district court, Southern District of Florida, ruled that the 1 January 1978 implementation date was invalid because it contradicted the date mandated by law.[37] The court ordered DHHS to determine whether or not the then-current Florida state Medicaid plan was in compliance with Section 249. The DHHS decision was to be made by 28 October 1977. If the Florida plan was not in compliance, the court ordered that Florida must submit a new plan for DHHS approval by 17 November 1977. When a Florida plan was acceptable to the department, its implementation date would be retroactive to 18 October 1977, the date of the district court ruling. As of 1 January 1978, the Florida program was still not in compliance with federal regulations for implementing Section 249. In this decision, the court decided not to rule on the question of retroactive reimbursement, based on reasonable-cost principles, back to the original 1 July 1976 implementation date for Section 249.

Federal courts in Illinois, Nebraska, and Wisconsin handed down similar decisions declaring the 1 January 1978 implementation date for Section 249 invalid.[38] The question of reasonable-cost-related payments retroactive to 1 July 1976 is critical, affecting the finances of both the state Medicaid programs and the long-term-care industry. As of September 1980, this question of retroactivity had not been decided in the courts.[39] This potentially devastating financial impact to state Medicaid programs was what Senator Bellmon had sought to avert with his amendment, which delayed the statutory implementation date of Section 249 and exempted state programs from liability for retroactive payments based on reasonable cost.

The ruling by the federal district court in Alabama, which stated that the financial inability of state programs to meet federal requirements does not excuse compliance, helps to explain the APWA's support for the Bellmon amendment. For those states that cannot meet the increased costs of compliance with Section 249, the only options are to raise additional revenues or to drop out of the Medicaid program. Since the APWA represents state Medicaid administrators, the reasons for its support of the Bellmon amendment become obvious.

Cost Analysis of Section 249

No cost-impact study was prepared for Section 249 during the formulation process, according to staff members for the Senate Finance Committee and the House Ways and Means Committee and officials in the Health Care Finance Administration of the DHHS. The legislative history makes clear that one reason for creating Section 249 was to increase the quality of the long-term care that Medicaid patients received. However, how much would this attempt to improve the quality of care cost? Would Section 249 generate benefits in excess of its costs? Without a cost study, this type of rational approach to decision making is impossible.

During 1972, the year Section 249 was before Congress, the nation's Medicaid program incurred a $1.47-billion expense for long-term care. Changing the reimbursement method for a program of this magnitude could have an immediate multimillion-dollar impact. Over a period of years this new policy could have a multibillion-dollar impact on the Medicaid program. Although it is a difficult task, the U.S. policymaking process can be faulted for failing to at least try to estimate the cost impact of Section 249.

The Medical Services Administration (MSA), an agency within the

DHHS, released in early 1976 a report titled *Inflation Impact Statement—Section 249 of PL 92–603*. This report estimated the cost impact of the new regulations for 1 July 1976 through 30 June 1977.[40]

To generate information for the analysis, a questionnaire was mailed to the states during September 1975. The state programs were asked to submit data on expenditures, patient days, and average payment rates for skilled-care and intermediate-care services. For the period 1 July 1976 through 30 June 1977, the states were first asked to project long-term-care costs assuming previous reimbursement methods were continued. Next, the states were asked to project costs for the same time period assuming compliance with Section 249. (The questionnaire included the proposed regulations for implementing Section 249 to guide the state officials in making their estimates.) The difference between these two sets of cost figures for the same time period were attributed, by the study, to the costs of complying with the new law for each state. The MSA analysis then totaled the compliance costs for all states, and this figure yielded the nationwide cost to the Medicaid program of complying with Section 249.

Forty-seven states responded to the survey. Of this total, thirty-four states predicted no cost impact because "they anticipated no change (in reimbursement practices) to be required—that they were now in compliance."[41] This claim of no cost impact by thirty-four states should be viewed with skepticism. (Later in the study, the MSA made upward revisions in its cost estimates due to its skepticism.) One year after these thirty-four states anticipated compliance, only two state programs had received DHHS approval for their reasonable-cost-related-reimbursement plans. Compliance with federal regulations for payments to nursing homes could increase Medicaid costs beyond the levels estimated by the states for the MSA cost-impact study.

Eleven states estimated that compliance with the federal regulations would increase skilled-nursing-facility costs in those states by a total of $56 million and intermediate-care-facility costs by $68 million. These eleven states estimated that for the time period 1 July 1976 through 30 June 1977, compliance with Section 249 would increase their total Medicaid expenditures for long-term care by $124 million (see appendix K).

For the five states that either did not respond to the questionnaire or were unable to estimate the cost impact of compliance with Section 249, the study reviewed each state's current reimbursement method and its current payment rates for long-term-care services. After analyzing the data for these state programs, the study concluded that only in Illinois would compliance with Section 249 have a cost impact.

The MSA analysis noted that "reimbursement rates for long-term-care services tend to be similar in contiguous states."[42] The estimates for skilled-care and intermediate-care services in Illinois were adjusted upward by this cost analysis to correspond with the costs for similar care in Wisconsin and Indiana. The MSA study concluded that compliance with federal regulations would add $28 million to Medicaid payments for nursing-home care in Illinois, raising the cost of implementing Section 249 to $152 million.

As mentioned earlier, the analysis recognized that many of the thirty-four states that anticipated no cost increase attributable to complying with Section 249, "may have underestimated the budgetary impact" of Section 249. Utilizing the same contiguous-state method used to calculate the cost increase for Illinois, the MSA study concluded that compliance in these thirty-four states "could easily add another $50 million to $150 million" to the total cost.

The "Inflation Impact Statement" concluded that the total cost of compliance to the Medicaid program would range from $202 million to $302 million for the time period 1 July 1976 through 30 June 1977. The scope of the study was limited because it assumed that this cost increase will only reflect higher prices for the same level of services that were delivered before the implementation of Section 249.[43] In other words, the study assumed that implementation of the new federal regulations would not change the long-term-care delivery system.

The analysis did not project possible increases in the quantity, or quality, of services delivered due to reasonable-cost-related reimbursement. If the quantity of services delivered increases, then this will add additional costs to the projected increases of $202–302 million. The important question to ask in this respect is: Will reimbursement based on reasonable cost of the services delivered encourage long-term-care institutions to deliver more services to patients? Average per diem costs measure the dollar value of the quantity of goods and services delivered to long-term-care patients.

Another change in the long-term-care system due to reasonable-cost reimbursement may be more patient days billable to the Medicaid program. Will state Medicaid-program compliance with Section 249 induce more long-term-care institutions to accept more Medicaid patients and for longer stays? Reasonable-cost-related reimbursement could make Medicaid patients as financially attractive to nursing-home operators as are private patients. Again, this possible change in the long-term-care system due to Section 249 would add to the total cost increase attributable to implementation.

Notes

1. Randall Ripley, William Moreland, and Richard Sinnreich, "Policy Making: A Conceptual Scheme," *American Politics Quarterly* 1 (January 1973):8.

2. Randall Ripley and Grace Franklin, *Congress, The Bureaucracy, and Public Policy* (Homewood, Ill.: Dorsey Press, 1976), pp. 5–7, 165–76. Also see Redford, *Democracy in the Administrative State* (New York: Oxford University Press, 1969), chapter IV, for a discussion of the subsystem model.

3. Ripley and Franklin, *Congress, The Bureaucracy, and Public Policy,* p. 5.

4. U.S., Congress, Senate, Committee on Finance, *Social Security Amendments of 1972,* 1972, Rept. 92–1230, p. 287.

5. Commerce Clearing House, "New Developments," *Medicare and Medicaid Guide,* para. 28, 835, Chicago: p. 9173.

6. Ibid.

7. Senator Carl T. Curtis, personal communication, 21 December 1978.

8. Jay Constantine, chief, Health Professional Staff, Senate Finance Committee, personal communication, 21 November 1978.

9. Interview with William Hermelin, administrator, Government Services, American Health Care Association, July 1978.

10. Laurance F. Lane, director for Public Policy, American Association of Homes for the Aging, personal communication, 5 February 1979. Reprinted with permission.

11. U.S., Congress, House of Representatives, Conference Committee, *Social Security Amendments of 1972,* 1972, Rept. 92–1605, 92nd Congress, 2nd sess., pp. 56–57.

12. U.S., Congress, Senate, *Congressional Record,* September 30, 1977, 92nd Congress, 2nd sess., p. 516009.

13. Dr. Paul Willging, acting director of the Medicaid Bureau, personal communication, 6 December 1978.

14. Congress, *Congressional Record,* 95th Congress, 1st sess., p. 516010.

15. Ibid.

16. Interview with Richard Nelson, press assistant to Congressman Mark Hanaford of California, June 1978.

17. Thomas Dye, *Understanding Public Policy,* 3rd ed. (Englewood Cliffs, N.J.: Prentice-Hall, 1978), pp. 23–25. For a detailed discussion of group theory, see David Truman, *The Government Process* (New York: Knopf, 1951).

18. Dye, *Understanding Public Policy,* p. 24.

19. "Congressional and Administrative News," *Laws* I(1972):1548–1747.

20. Commerce Clearing House, "New Developments," *Medicare and Medicaid Guide* para. 28, 712, ꜰ 10507.

21. Senate, *Social Security Amendments of 1972,* 1972, Rept. 92–1230, 92nd Congress, 2nd sess., p. 287.

22. Dr. Paul Willging, acting director of the Medicaid program, personal communication, 6 December 1978.

23. Commerce Clearing House, "State Plan Requirements," *Medicare and Medicaid Guide,* para. 14723, pp. 63793–794.

24. Senate, *Social Security Amendments of 1972,* 1972, Rept. 92–1230, 92nd Congress, 2nd sess., p. 287.

25. Commerce Clearing House, "New Developments," para. 28, 835, p. 9178.

26. Interview with William Hermelin, American Health Care Association, July 1978.

27. Ibid.

28. *American Health Care Association, Inc.* v. *Califano,* U.S. District Court, District of Columbia, 7 December 1977, in Commerce Clearing House, *Medicare and Medicaid Guide,* para. 28, 684, pp. 10395–398.

29. *American Health Care Association* v. *Califano, Medicare and Medicaid Guide,* para. 28, 684, p. 10396.

30. Ibid., pp. 10396–397.

31. Senate, *Social Security Amendments of 1972,* 92nd Congress, 2nd sess., pp. 287–88.

32. *American Health Care Association* v. *Califano, Medicare and Medicaid Guide,* para. 28, 684, p. 10397.

33. Ibid.

34. *Federal Register* 43, no. 25, 6 February 1978, 4861–64.

35. "Cases Argued and Determined in the United States District Court," *Federal Supplement* 433(1 December 1977):1325.

36. Carl Wendorf, "State's Reimbursement for Long-Term Care Must Be on a Reasonable-Cost-Related Basis," *Hospitals* 51(1 December 1977): 38.

37. Commerce Clearing House, *Medicare and Medicaid Guide,* para. 28, 709, pp. 10502–503.

38. Ibid., pp. 10504–513.

39. Interview with Marc Levin, American Health Care Association, 24 September 1980.

40. U.S., Department of Health, Education, and Welfare, Medical Services Administration, *Inflationary Impact Statement? Section 249 of PL 92–603,"* 1976.

41. Ibid., p. 6.

42. Ibid., p. 7.

43. Ibid., p. 2.

6

Summary and Conclusions

This study has analyzed the impact that Medicaid reimbursement practices have had on the cost and utilization of skilled and intermediate care to elderly Americans. The public sector, through the Medicare and Medicaid programs, has become the primary purchaser of long-term care. During 1976 all levels of U.S. government financed 55 percent of the nursing-home care purchased in this country (see table 1–1). Payments to long-term-care facilities absorbed an estimated 44 percent of total Medicaid spending during 1980, making this the largest Medicaid expenditure category (see table 1–3). Since 1972, Medicaid expenditures for long-term care in Virginia have increased from $4.4 million to $102.8 million in 1977 (see table 1–5). Every year nursing-home care consumes a larger share of the Medicaid pie.

Table 6–1 projects the future growth of the U.S. population, 65 years and over. The enormous burden of this increasingly older population on the Social Security system and the Medicare program has been widely discussed in public-policy circles. However, the danger in these demographic changes to the Medicaid program has not been as thoroughly discussed. Medicaid expenditures for nursing-home care will skyrocket as the American population becomes increasingly older. The dramatic growth that has already occurred in Medicaid payments for long-term care is merely a prelude to the future cost explosion when demographic changes add new pressures to the upward-cost spiral.

Table 6–1
U.S. Population Projections
(*millions*)

Year	Total Population	65 and over	Percentage 65 and over
1970	204.8	20.2	9.9
1985	229.2	25.3	11.0
2000	249.0	28.1	11.3
2025	271.4	42.4	15.6
2050	273.2	43.8	16.0

Source: U.S., National Science Foundation, *Economies of a Stationary Population: Implications for Older Americans,* NSF/RA–77021, 1977, table 4, p. 17.

One purpose of this research was to catalogue and describe the national Medicaid reimbursement system from 1973 to 1977. This payment structure was then analyzed to determine what impact, if any, the different reimbursement methods have had on the cost and utilization of nursing-home care. Do payment methods exist that can reduce the cost of care to the Medicaid program without adversely affecting Medicaid patients' access to long-term care? As the number of elderly Americans increases, which increases the consumer base for nursing-home care, the discovery of cost-saving reimbursement methods becomes even more important in the effort to minimize public spending.

The Profit versus Nonprofit Debate

As discussed in chapter 2, many critics of the long-term-care industry attribute the problems relating to cost and quality of care to the profit motive. Most nursing-home care in the United States is delivered by proprietary facilities. According to some critics, proprietary institutions make excessive profits while delivering inadequate patient care. Does the profit motive add to the cost spiral for nursing-home care? Should proprietary ownership of nursing homes be phased out as the AFL-CIO recommends?

Profits

This study analyzed long-term-care profits and the impact that type of ownership has had on the price and quality of care. Table 2-1 compared the profitability of the United States' leading long-term-care corporations with other U.S. industries. Over the seven-year period surveyed, the profit margins for the long-term-care index developed for this analysis were always lower than the average profit margins for U.S. industry in general. The highest profit margin for the nursing-home index was 3.2 percent in 1977; the lowest profit margin for the total industry composite was 4.8 percent during the recession of 1975. Table 2-1 clearly demonstrates that the large long-term-care chains are not making excessive profits as their critics have charged. The potential to earn a profit is what attracts capital into an industry, causing production and output to expand. The low profitability of nursing-home companies, relative to other U.S. industry, may explain the shortage of long-term-care beds in some areas of the United States. Greater rewards can be earned by investing resources in other opportunities.

Four Seasons Nursing Centers, Inc., presents an interesting example of capital movement. Far from being highly profitable, this once-major nursing-home chain filed for protection under the bankruptcy laws in the early

1970s. In 1972 the company reorganized under the new name of Anta Corporation, with Four Seasons Nursing Centers as its principal business. The
first major moves of the reorganized company were to sell many of its
nursing centers and to diversify into other industries. In 1979 Anta had an
aluminum-products division, a plastic-packaging division, and a drilling,
oil, and gas division, as well as the Four Seasons Nursing Centers.[1] If
profitability and return on investment were high, as the critics of proprietary nursing homes have charged, it seems unlikely that Anta would have
shifted its capital to these other industries. Capital flows to areas that offer
the greatest promise for long-term profits, not away from profit-maximiz-
ing opportunities. During the first three months of 1979, Anta sold two
additional nursing centers in Texas, indicating that higher profits can be
made with that capital in uses other than nursing homes. Anta is also
increasing the percentage of private patients in its remaining nursing-home
centers, indicating the current reluctance of the industry to accept Medicaid
patients due to lower reimbursement rates.

Costs

Another important question in the profit-versus-nonprofit debate concerns
the prices of skilled and intermediate care. Do proprietary facilities charge
higher prices for the care they deliver compared to nonprofit institutions?
Given the expected future cost spiral, would the phasing out of proprietary
nursing homes reduce the upward-cost pressures?

A study of Massachusetts nursing homes for 1966 concluded that
proprietary nursing homes were usually less expensive than nonprofit
homes. A 1966 study of Minnesota long-term-care facilities revealed that
the type of ownership had no significant affect on the cost of care. A study
of Virginia nursing homes for 1974 revealed that proprietary institutions
delivered care at a lower per diem cost than nonprofit facilities, although
the difference was not statistically significant.

Based on the studies surveyed, either no difference exists in the prices
charged to deliver care between types of ownership, or if a difference does
exist, the profit-seeking homes are less expensive. Phasing the profit motive
out of the delivery of long-term care to reduce Medicaid expenditures would
not achieve the desired result. It would more likely increase Medicaid expenditures for nursing-home care.

Quality

Chapter 2 also reviewed studies that explored for differences in the quality
of care delivered by type of ownership. Does a difference exist in the quality

of care delivered by profit and nonprofit nursing homes? The major conclusion of the studies surveyed was that there were no significant differences in the services delivered by type of ownership. If these services delivered are reliable proxy measures for the quality of care, then there is no difference in the quality of care delivered by proprietary and nonprofit institutions. Removing the profit motive from nursing homes would not necessarily improve the quality of care delivered to patients.

The major conclusion of this analysis concerning type of ownership is that the profit motive should not be removed from the long-term-care industry. Phasing out proprietary facilities would not necessarily improve the quality of care delivered, and it probably would increase the costs of care.

Rather than remove the profit motive, incentives should be built into the Medicaid system to use the profit motive to increase efficiency in the delivery of care. The challenge to the administrators of the Medicaid program is to develop reimbursement methods to harness the profit motive in order to increase efficiency, while safeguarding the Medicaid patients from abuse and neglect. The quality of care delivered to the elderly should be a concern equal to that of cost reduction. Economic efficiency does not mean simply reducing costs. It means reducing costs while maintaining the quality of the care delivered. With increased future emphasis on cost reduction, Medicaid administrators have the primary responsibility to protect patients from the wolves of the nursing-home industry.

The Medicaid Reimbursement System

Chapter 3 explored the Medicaid reimbursement system for nursing-home care in the attempt to discover methods that could harness the profit motive to encourage the efficient delivery of care. Three major methods have been used by the state Medicaid programs to determine the amount of reimbursement to long-term-care facilities. These methods are: reasonable-cost-related reimbursement, fixed-rate reimbursement, and negotiated-rate reimbursement.

In chapter 3 five policy goals for a reimbursement method relating to efficiency and the quality of care were established. The fixed-rate and negotiated-rate methods both contain incentives to minimize costs. When these methods are used, the long-term-care institution is paid a flat per diem fee for each type of care delivered. The profit to the nursing home is the difference between the per diem rate and the incurred costs. Unlike reasonable-cost-related reimbursement, these methods provide the incentive to the health-care facility to deliver only needed services and to innovate in order to lower the costs of delivery.

When the reimbursement rate is a function of the actual cost of care delivered, incentives for reducing costs are minimized. If state Medicaid programs have complete retroactive reimbursement of total incurred costs, then the payment method itself can be a disincentive to minimizing the costs of delivering care.

The reasonable-cost-related-reimbursement method provides a greater incentive to deliver higher-quality health care than do the other methods. When payment is a function of the actual cost of care delivered, the nursing home has the incentive to deliver all reimbursable services to Medicaid patients. The possibility of fraud still exists, even with the reasonable-cost method, making it necessary for Medicaid officials to monitor operations to guarantee that billed services are in fact delivered to patients.

Potential disincentives exist for delivering high-quality care in states using the negotiated-rate and fixed-rate methods of reimbursement. Since profit to nursing homes in these states is the difference between the per diem fee and the actual cost of delivering care, the danger exists that skilled-care and intermediate-care facilities will reduce the quantity and quality of services delivered. Again, Medicaid officials have the reponsibility to monitor the services delivered to guarantee that cost cutting does not lead to undue reduction in the quality of care.

Chapter 4 analyzed reimbursement methods from a statistical perspective to determine what impact reasonable-cost-related, fixed-rate, and nego- tiated-rate reimbursement have had on the cost and utilization of nursing- home care. The major findings about the delivery of skilled care support the contention that the reasonable-cost-related-payment method does not contain incentives to minimize costs. From 1973 to 1977 the average per diem cost of skilled care in states using the reasonable-cost-related method was consistently higher than in states using the other two methods. In three of the five years, the difference in average per diem cost for skilled care among the reimbursement methods was statistically significant. States using the negotiated-rate method always had the lowest average per diem cost for skilled care during this time span.

Only if the quality of the skilled care delivered in the states using the different reimbursement methods is assumed equal, and this study does not make this assumption, can the negotiated-rate method be called the most- efficient payment method. Assessing the quality of care, however, is beyond the scope of this study. Looking at cost alone, the major conclusion con- cerning reimbursement methods is that states using the negotiated-rate method consistently had the lowest per diem rates for skilled care, and states using the reasonable-cost-related method consistently had the highest rates.

The method of reimbursement also affected the utilization of skilled care by Medicaid patients. States using the negotiated-rate method consistently had fewer Medicaid patients per 1,000 of their elderly population receiving skilled care than did states using the other two payment methods. The conclusion drawn was that due to the low payment rates for skilled care in these states, skilled-care facilities reduced the number of Medicaid patients they accepted. Not surprisingly, states using the negotiated-rate method of reimbursement had the highest utilization rates for intermediate care. These conclusions suggest that patients refused by skilled-care homes in states using the negotiated-rate method were placed in intermediate-care facilities. If Medicaid payment rates are insufficient to cover the costs of providing skilled care, then skilled-care facilities in these states will either refuse to accept Medicaid patients to make room for higher-paying private patients or not even develop skilled-care beds. No statistically significant differences existed in average per diem costs among reimbursement methods for intermediate care.

The reimbursement method used can affect the price, quality, and access to long-term care. If, in the attempt to reduce long-term-care expenditures, state Medicaid programs establish inadequate per diem rates, then not only will the quality of care be jeopardized but also nursing-home care might not be available to Medicaid patient.

Impacts of PL 92–603 (Section 249)

During 1972 the Senate Finance Committee was concerned that Medicaid reimbursement methods could have a negative impact on the long-term-care system. The concern was that the wide range of reimbursement practices used by the state programs to pay for skilled and intermediate care may have resulted in some states paying too much for care and other states paying too little "to support the quality of care Medicaid patients are expected to need and receive."[2] The Senate Finance Committee recognized the potential danger that inadequate per diem rates might cause nursing homes either to deliver inadequate care or refuse to accept Medicaid patients.

The committee's objective was to standardize the reimbursement method nationwide and to establish a system that would promote efficiency and maintain the quality of care. The policy response was to require that all state Medicaid programs reimburse long-term-care facilities on a reasonable-cost-related basis, effective 1 July 1976. Acute-care hospitals were already reimbursed at that time on a reasonable-cost basis by both the Medicare and Medicaid programs. This precedent was the legislative ancestor of Section 249. Chapter 5 detailed the development of Section 249 as well as the delay in implementation and the resulting legal challenges.

How much will it cost the Medicaid program to switch to the reasonable-cost-related system as required by PL 92–603 (Section 249)? No cost estimate was made during the policy-formulation process of Section 249. During 1976 the MSA, an agency within the DHHS, estimated the total cost of compliance at between $202 million and $302 million for the period from 1 July 1976 through 30 June 1977. Chapter 5 reviewed and critiqued that analysis. The major criticism of that study is that it projected only cost changes and did not consider what impact the new law would have on utilization. If reasonable-cost-related reimbursement would increase per diem–payment rates, as the MSA study predicted, would the willingness of long-term-care facilities to accept Medicaid patients be increased. The statistical analysis in chapter 4 revealed that states using the reasonable-cost-related reimbursement method do have higher average scores for the utilization indexes, indicating that Section 249 will increase Medicaid expenditures beyond the 1976 estimate issued by the MSA.

A staff report prepared for the Senate Finance Committee in March 1979 estimated that eliminating Section 249 would save the state Medicaid programs a total of $250 million per year.[3] Edward A. Beck, the legislative assistant to Senator Harry F. Byrd, Jr., of Virginia, stated that this estimate was made after a review of the current program and consultation with the General Accounting Office (GAO).[4] The Congressional Budget Office (CBO) also made a similar cost estimate for Section 249 according to the legislative assistant.

Prospective and Retrospective Reimbursement

Another long-term-care-reimbursement issue concerns the debate over prospective- and retrospective-rate setting. The per diem–reimbursement fee can be calculated either on a prospective or retrospective basis. The prospective method determines the payment rate for each class of care prior to the delivery of care. The retrospective method determines the per diem rate for each type of care after the care is delivered to the patient, based on incurred costs. Chapter 3 presented the issues relating to this prospective versus retrospective debate. The major argument for prospective reimbursement is the hypothesis that this method promotes cost containment in the delivery of care. The principal argument against prospective reimbursement is the charge that it could adversely affect the utilization of care by Medicaid patients.

The statistical analysis of prospective and retrospective reimbursement presented in chapter 4 demonstrated that no statistically significant difference exists in outcomes for the utilization indexes between the two rate-setting methods. The conclusion is that prospective reimbursement does not have an adverse affect on Medicaid patients' access to long-term care.

The statistical analysis also revealed that significant differences exist in the average per diem–payment rates for skilled and intermediate care paid by state Medicaid programs using the two different techniques. Prospective-rate determination was associated with lower average per diem costs than was retrospective-rate setting. This study concludes that the prospective method contains incentives to encourage health-care providers to minimize the delivery costs of care. As the percentage of elderly Americans increases dramatically during the remainder of this century, and given the outlook for continued inflation in the U.S. economy, prospective-rate setting should be used by state Medicaid programs to minimize nursing-home expenditures.

Recommended Prospective System

To contain rising long-term-care costs in the future, the Medicaid program should move away from a reimbursement system that repays allowable costs of care on a retrospective basis. This method does not encourage efficiency in the delivery of nursing-home care since the institutions receive payments based on their incurred costs. Prospective reimbursement offers the promise of introducing cost containment incentives into the delivery of nursing-home care.

The prospective rate should be based upon the actual cost of delivering a particular classification of care. This basis would satisfy the federal reimbursement requirement established for state Medicaid programs by PL 92–603 (Section 249). The first step in this proposed payment system would be to define the various classifications of care, differentiated by the nursing services and other health care delivered. Next, all long-term-care facilities within the state or geographic subdivision of the state would be grouped into these classifications. An average cost of care for each classification would be calculated based upon the actual costs from the previous year. The prospective rate would then be determined for the new fiscal period as some function of this classification mean (mean plus X percent).

If the nursing home can deliver the care at a cost below this fixed per diem fee, then the facility would be allowed to keep a varying percentage of the difference as an efficiency incentive. The exact percentage would be based on the institutions's score on a quality-of-care index. This index would measure the nursing home's compliance with Medicaid-certification standards for quality and safety. The higher the long-term-care facility's score on the index, the larger the percentage of the difference between actual cost and the prospective-payment rate it could keep as an incentive bonus.

If the nursing home did not meet a minimally acceptable level on this quality-of-care index, it would then have to return the entire difference between the fixed payment and its incurred costs. Extreme offenders of the quality-of-care index would be penalized through graduated reductions in their reimbursement as their index scores declined.

Retroactive adjustment of the prospective rate would be allowed to prevent unforeseen cost increases from reducing the quality of care. However, future incentive bonuses would be reduced to repay any retrospective cost adjustments. This proposed prospective-rate method would have incentives for both cost efficiency and the delivery of high-quality care.

Conclusion

The population projections presented in this study clearly indicate that long-term-care expenses will skyrocket in future years. These dramatic cost increases will place a heavy financial burden on the state Medicaid programs, which are the primary purchasers of nursing-home care in the United States.

To minimize these future costs this study advocates that the profit motive be harnessed to provide incentives to minimize the costs of care while maintaining or increasing the quality of care delivered. A prospective-reimbursement system can provide the incentives to profit-seeking nursing homes to minimize costs. Linking the per diem fee to a quality-of-care index would guard against the danger of sacrificing quality to increase profit. The higher a nursing home's score on a quality-of-care index, the larger the percentage of the difference between the prospective rate and the actual cost of care the long-term-care facility would be allowed to keep.

The thrust of this analysis has been to discover reimbursement methods that can provide incentives to the profit-seeking nursing home to efficiently deliver high-quality care to Medicaid patients. This research has focused on the nonhuman elements of nursing-home care—primarily the statistical impact that reimbursement has had on cost and utilization. A danger of statistical analysis is that the analyst can forget that these services are delivered to people. Concerns for cost efficiency may overshadow concern for the elderly people who are placed in these health-care institutions.

Concern for the human needs of the institutionalized elderly should at least equal, if not exceed, public concern for cost efficiency. Ideally, ways will be found to give these forgotten Americans a sense of meaning and purpose in our society. As an example, a recent public-service message on television, designed to encourage the community to accept the elderly back into life, has shown elderly people nursing and rocking institutionalized infants. This symbiotic relationship provides the warmth of human touch and affection to the forgotten infants and allows the forgotten elderly to again contribute part of themselves; they are needed again.

Cost reduction out of necessity will become a major concern to Medicaid officials. Of equal concern, however, should be the patients and the quality of care they receive. Since nursing-home patients cannot always act in their own best interests to guarantee the quality of care they receive, government, as the major purchaser of care, must assume this responsibility.

Notes

1. U.S., Department of Health, Education, and Welfare, Social Security Administration, *Research and Statistics Note* 22 December 1976, p. 3.

2. U.S., Congress, Senate, Committee on Finance, *Social Security Amendments of 1972,* 1972, Rept. 92–1230, 92nd Congress, 2nd sess., p. 287.

3. U.S., Congress, Senate, Committees on Finance, *Health Care Cost Containment and Other Proposals,* Committee Print 96–9, 20 March 1979, p. 35.

4. Edward A. Beck, legislative assistant to Senator Harry F. Byrd, Jr., of Virginia to Robert J. Buchanan, 6 July 1979.

Appendix A
Leading
Long-Term-Care
Companies

Revenue and Income (Loss) Data for 1973–1979
(thousands of dollars)

Long-Term-Care Chains	Revenues	Net Income
1973		
Hill Haven	47.449	1,689
Beverly Enterprises	42,893	(3,083)
National Health	39,471	1,639
Unicare	36,508	(1,363)
Aid, Inc.	50,486	401
Monterey Life Systems	24,878	1,073
Continental Care	12,940	518
Manor Care	12,187	714
American Medical Affiliates	11,636	193
Gold Medallion	16,216	426
Guardian	5,156	315
Medicalodges	4,533	229
Care Corporation	2,830	95
Total	307,183	2,846

Profit as Percentage of Sales: 0.0092

1974		
Hill Haven	57,888	1,162
Beverly Enterprises	50,870	(5,100)
National Health	55,880	333
Unicare	35,314	1,018
Aid, Inc.	71,588	706
Monterey Life Systems	27,084	858
Continental Care	17,299	925
Manor Care	16,047	558
American Medical Affiliates	12,994	196
Gold Medallion	16,549	46
Guardian	7,410	359
Medicalodges	5,970	261
Care Corporation	3,243	125
Total	378,136	1,447

Profit as Percentage of Sales: 0.0038

Long-Term-Care Chains	Revenues	Net Income
1975		
Hill Haven	78,166	928
Beverly Enterprises	56,889	563
National Health	61,279	(1,462)
Unicare	39,424	1,333
Aid, Inc.	85,046	2,237
Monterey Life Systems	29,018	(780)
Continental Care	22,220	679
Manor Care	20,756	514
American Medical Affiliates	16,501	1,092
Gold Medallion	15,579	(554)
Guardian	9,406	334
Medicalodges	9,392	272
Care Corporation	20,483	597
Total	464,159	5,753

Profit as Percentage of Sales: 0.012

1976		
Hill Haven	97,580	1,283
Beverly Enterprises	66,670	(1,548)
National Health	64,448	611
Unicare	40,612	1,850
Aid, Inc.	108,408	3,305
Monterey Life Systems	N.A.	N.A.
Continental Care	N.A.	N.A.
Manor Care	30,321	1,358
American Medical Affiliates	17,765	663
Gold Medallion	19,829	489
Guardian	N.A.	N.A.
Medicalodges	10.013	291
Care Corporation	22,555	743
Total	478,201	9,045

Profit as Percentage of Sales: 0.019

1977		
Hill Haven	121,705	2,116
Beverly Enterprises	81,331	3,534
National Health	68,886	1,124
Unicare	50,597	1,521
Aid, Inc.	149,448	4,114
Monterey Life Systems	N.A.	N.A.
Continental Care	N.A.	N.A.
Manor Care	30,668	1,796

Long-Term-Care Chains	Revenues	Net Income
American Medical Affiliates	25,016	647
Gold Medallion	21,191	276
Guardian	N.A.	N.A.
Medicalodges	12,079	308
Care Corporation	26,887	764
Total	587,808	16,200

Profit as Percentage of Sales: 0.028

1978

Hill Haven	155,963	2,998
Beverly Enterprises	139,868	5,832
National Health	75,678	1,613
Unicare	66,445	1,703
Aid, Inc.	(acquired by INA Corporation)	
Monterey Life Systems	N.A.	N.A.
Continental Care	N.A.	N.A.
Manor Care	36,886	1,796
American Medical Affiliates	30,592	1,022
Gold Medallion	23,624	517
Guardian	N.A.	N.A.
Medicalodges	17,527	394
Care Corporation	29,518	1,028
Total	576,101	16,903

Profit as Percentage of Sales: 0.029

1979

Hill Haven	200,858	4,598
Beverly Enterprises	173,500	5,879
National Health	83,136	2,058
Unicare	82,644	1,206
Aid, Inc.	(acquired by INA Corporation)	
Monterey Life Systems	N.A.	N.A.
Continental Care	N.A.	N.A.
Manor Care	47,261	2,525
American Medical Affiliates	32,492	195
Gold Medallion	28,092	50
Guardian	N.A.	N.A.
Medicalodges	N.A.	N.A
Care Corporation	32,853	1,125
Total	680,836	17,636

Profit as Percentage of Sales: 0.026

Source: Data obtained from each company's *10-K Report*.
Note: N.A. means the information was not available.

Appendix B
State Listing of Reimbursement Method and Average Per Diem Cost for 1973–1977

Unless otherwise noted, information on the type of reimbursement method used in each state for both skilled-care facilities and intermediate-care facilities was obtained from individual state Medicaid plans on file with the U.S. Department of Health and Human Services in Washington, D.C.

Medicaid Reimbursement: Method and Cost

Year	Reimbursement Method		Average Per Diem Cost	
	Skilled-care Facility	Intermediate-Care Facility	Skilled-Care Facility	Intermediate-Care Facility
Alabama				
1977	Reasonable cost with ceiling	Reasonable cost with ceiling	$21.16[c]	$18.03[c]
1976	Reasonable cost with ceiling	Reasonable cost with ceiling	20.00[c]	17.85[c]
1975	Reasonable cost with ceiling	Reasonable cost with ceiling	15.49[b]	13.77[b]
1974	N.A.	N.A.	11.28[e]	9.30[e]
1973	N.A.	N.A.	9.67[f]	10.28[f]
Alaska				
1977	Reasonable cost	Reasonable cost 10 percent less than skilled-care facility	N.A.	N.A.
1976	Reasonable cost	Reasonable cost 10 percent less than skilled-care facility	60.95[b]	40.12[b]
1975	Cost Settlement[1]	Cost Settlement[1] 10 percent less than skilled-care facility	50.79[b]	33.43[b]
1974	Cost Settlement[1]	Cost Settlement[1] 10 percent less than skilled-care facility	31.07[e]	24.06[e]
1973	N.A.	N.A.	24.23[f]	22.42[f]

107

	Reimbursement Method		Average Per Diem Cost	
Year	Skilled-Care Facility	Intermediate-Care Facility	Skilled-Care Facility	Intermediate-Care Facility
Arkansas				
1977	Fixed Rate [a]	Fixed Rate [a]	16.00 [b]	$11.48[b]
1976	Fixed Rate [a]	Fixed Rate [a]	16.00[b]	11.48[b]
1975	Fixed Rate [a]	Fixed Rate [a]	16.00[b]	11.48[b]
1974	Fixed Rate [a]	Fixed Rate [a]	9.57 [e]	7.23 [e]
1973	Fixed Rate [a]	Fixed Rate [a]	8.98 [f]	6.82[f]
California				
1977	Fixed Rate [a]	Fixed Rate [a]	24.81 [a]	19.72[a]
1976	Fixed Rate [a]	Fixed Rate [a]	22.77 [a]	17.64[a]
1975	Fixed Rate [a]	Fixed Rate [a]	19.81[a]	15.96[a]
1974	Fixed Rate [a]	Fixed Rate [a]	17.81[a]	14.59[a]
1973	Fixed Rate [a]	Fixed Rate [a]	16.78[a]	10.60[a]
Colorado				
1977	Actual audited costs for each skilled-care facility	Actual audited costs for each intermediate-care facility	17.27 [b]	16.41 [b]
1976	Actual audited costs for each skilled-care facility	Actual audited costs for each intermediate-care facility	16.45 [b]	15.62[b]
1975	Actual audited costs for each skilled-care facility	Actual audited costs for each intermediate-care facility	15.23 [b]	14.88[b]
1974	Actual audited costs for each skilled-care facility	Actual audited costs for each intermediate-care facility	N.A.	N.A.
1973	Actual audited costs for each skilled-care facility	Actual audited costs for each intermediate-care facility	N.A.	N.A.
Connecticut				
1977	Reasonable cost with ceiling	Reasonable cost with ceiling	26.34 [b]	15.16 [b]
1976	Reasonable cost with ceiling	Reasonable cost with ceiling	24.85[b]	14.30 [b]
1975	Unaudited cost plus 5 percent [a]	Unaudited cost plus 5 percent [a]	23.00[b]	13.25 [b]
1974	Fixed Rate [a]	Fixed Rate [a]	15.37 [e]	N.A.
1973	Fixed Rate [a]	Fixed Rate [a]	15.65 [f]	N.A.

Year	Reimbursement Method		Average Per Diem Cost	
	Skilled-Care Facility	Intermediate-Care Facility	Skilled-Care Facility	Intermediate-Care Facility
Delaware				
1977	Reasonable cost	Reasonable cost	25.85[c]	25.85[c]
1976	Cost plus 6 percent[2]	Reasonable cost[2]	22.00[c]	18.17[c]
1975	Cost plus 6 percent[a]	Cost plus 6 percent[a]	12.90[b]	18.41[b]
1974	Cost plus 6 percent[a]	Cost plus 6 percent[a]	12.82[e]	11.37[e]
1973	Cost plus 6 percent[a]	Cost plus 6 percent[a]	12.79[f]	4.54[f]
Florida				
1977	Lowest of: 1. Flat rate— $630/month 2. Reasonable cost[3] 3. Rate for private care	Lowest of: 1. Flat rate— $560; $500/ month 2. Percent of skilled-care facility rate 3. Rate for private care	15.50[b]	11.62[b]
1976	Lowest of: 1. Flat rate— $630/month 2. Reasonable cost 3. Rate for private care	Lowest of: 1. Flat rate— $560; $500/ month 2. Percent of skilled-care facility rate 3. Rate for private care	15.01[b]	11.62[b]
1975	Lowest of: 1. Flat rate— $550/month 2. Reasonable cost 3. Rate for private care	Lowest of: Flat rate— $450/month 2. Reasonable cost 3. Rate for private care	13.80[b]	10.25[b]
1974	Lowest of: 1. Flat rate— $550/month 2. Reasonable cost 3. Rate for private care	Lowest of: 1. Flat rate— $375/month 2. Reasonable cost 3. Rate for private care	10.80[e]	7.75[e]
1973	N.A.	N.A.	9.43[f]	6.46[f]
Georgia				
1977	Reasonable cost	Reasonable cost	15.00[b]	14.10[b]
1976	Reasonable cost	Reasonable cost	14.82[b]	13.96[b]
1975	Reasonable cost	Reasonable cost	14.39[b]	13.65[b]
1974	N.A.	N.A.	9.97[e]	7.50[e]
1973	N.A.	N.A.	9.85[f]	6.89[f]

Year	Reimbursement Method		Average Per Diem Cost	
	Skilled-Care Facility	Intermediate-Care Facility	Skilled-Care Facility	Intermediate-Care Facility
Hawaii				
1977	Reasonable cost	Negotiated[4]	41.30[c]	39.05[c]
1976	Reasonable cost	Negotiated	37.36[c]	34.45[c]
1975	Reasonable cost	Negotiated	29.11[b]	18.61[b]
1974	Reasonable cost	Negotiated	23.11[e]	18.15[e]
1973	N.A.	N.A.	19.19[f]	N.A.
Idaho				
1977	Reasonable cost	Reasonable cost	20.77[a]	18.09[b]
1976	Reasonable cost	Reasonable cost	17.79[b]	16.14[b]
1975	Reasonable cost	Reasonable cost	17.45[b]	15.23[b]
1974	Reasonable cost	Reasonable cost	10.04[e]	5.27[e]
1973	N.A.	N.A.	8.87[f]	N.A.
Illinois				
1977	Fixed rate	Fixed rate	22.32[c]	15.63[c]
1976	Fixed rate	Fixed rate	21.55[c]	15.37[c]
1975	Fixed rate	Fixed rate	18.84[c]	16.08[c]
	Fixed rate	Fixed rate	15.50[e]	13.93[e]
1973	N.A.	N.A.	14.35[f]	8.14[f]
Indiana				
1977	Cost related	Cost related	25.21[a]	15.27[a]
1976	Cost related	Cost related	24.15[a]	14.38[a]
1975	Cost related	Cost related	21.42[a]	12.57[a]
1974	Cost related	Cost related	19.96[e]	11.60[e]
1973	Cost related	N.A.	N.A.	N.A.
Iowa				
1977	Reasonable cost	Reasonable cost	30.07[c]	19.60[c]
1976	Reasonable cost	Reasonable cost	23.46[c]	17.75[c]
1975	Reasonable cost[a]	Reasonable cost[a]	18.54[d]	9.62[d]
1974	Reasonable cost[a]	Reasonable cost[a]	18.38[e]	8.04[e]
1973	Reasonable cost[a]	Reasonable cost[a]	19.12[f]	7.50[f]
Kansas				
1977	Reasonable cost[a]	Reasonable cost[a]	24.23[a]	16.10[a]
1976	Reasonable cost[a]	Reasonable cost[a]	15.39[b]	12.01[b]
1975	Reasonable cost[a]	Reasonable cost[a]	14.16[b]	11.75[b]
1974	Reasonable cost[a]	Reasonable cost[a]	8.86[e]	5.74[e]
1973	[5]	[5]	7.97[f]	6.14[f]

Year	Reimbursement Method		Average Per Diem Cost	
	Skilled-Care Facility	Intermediate-Care Facility	Skilled-Care Facility	Intermediate-Care Facility
Kentucky				
1977	Reasonable cost	Fixed rate	31.57 [c]	18.43 [c]
1976	Reasonable rate	Fixed rate	29.37 [c]	17.30 [c]
1975	Reasonable cost	Fixed rate	26.49 [b]	11.57 [b]
1974	Reasonable cost	Fixed rate	17.63 [e]	8.38 [e]
1973	Reasonable cost	Fixed rate	16.72 [f]	8.19 [f]
Louisiana				
1977	Reasonable cost [6]	Reasonable cost [6]	21.06 [c]	12.52 [c]
1976	Negotiated rate [6] Reasonable cost	Negotiated rate [6] Reasonable cost	17.69 [c]	11.23 [c]
1975	Negotiated rate	Negotiated rate	12.60 [b]	11.74 [b]
1974	Negotiated rate	Negotiated rate	8.94 [e]	8.49 [e]
1973	Negotiated rate	Negotiated rate	9.11 [f]	7.89 [f]
Maine				
1977	Reasonable cost	Reasonable cost	56.31 [a]	22.95 [a]
1976	Reasonable cost	Reasonable cost	47.77 [a]	21.80 [a]
1975	Reasonable cost	N.A.	N.A.	N.A.
1974	Reasonable cost	N.A.	N.A.	N.A.
1973	Reasonable cost	N.A.	N.A.	N.A.
Maryland				
1977	Cost plus profit	Cost plus profit	19.86 [c]	17.56 [c]
1976	Cost plus profit	Cost plus profit	18.40 [c]	16.49 [c]
1975	Cost plus profit	Cost plus profit	16.74 [d]	14.53 [d]
1974	Cost plus profit	Cost plus profit	15.50 [e]	13.72 [e]
1973	N.A.	N.A.	14.10 [f]	12.27 [f]
Massachusetts				
1977	Reasonable cost [a]	Reasonable cost [a]	N.A.	N.A.
1976	Reasonable cost [a]	Reasonable cost [a]	N.A.	N.A.
1975	Reasonable cost [a]	Reasonable cost [a]	21.19 [d]	16.30 [d]
1974	Reasonable cost [a]	Reasonable cost [a]	N.A.	N.A.
1973	Reasonable cost [a]	Reasonable cost [a]	N.A.	N.A.
Michigan				
1977	Fixed rate	Fixed rate	20.30 [c]	18.90 [c]
1976	Fixed rate	Fixed rate	19.14 [c]	17.62 [c]
1975	Fixed rate	Fixed rate	18.84 [d]	16.08 [d]
1974	Fixed rate	Fixed rate	17.22 [e]	13.93 [e]
1973	Fixed rate	Fixed rate	N.A.	N.A.

	Reimbursement Method		Average Per Diem Cost	
Year	Skilled-Care Facility	Intermediate-Care Facility	Skilled-Care Facility	Intermediate-Care Facility
Minnesota				
1977	Reasonable cost	Reasonable cost	25.83 [c]	N.A.
1976	Reasonable cost	Reasonable cost	23.02 [c]	N.A.
1975	Reasonable cost	Reasonable cost	18.44 [d]	13.26 [d]
1974	Reasonable cost	Reasonable cost	10.87 [e]	7.34 [e]
1973	N.A.	N.A.	13.54 [f]	8.89 [f]
Mississippi				
1977	Reasonable cost	Reasonable cost	24.25 [c]	21.50 [c]
1976	Fixed rate	Fixed rate	15.86 [b]	12.90 [b]
1975	Fixed rate	Fixed rate	14.04 [b]	12.83 [b]
1974	Fixed rate	Fixed rate	11.80 [e]	10.58 [e]
1973	Fixed rate	Fixed rate	10.21 [f]	6.92 [f]
Missouri				
1977	Reasonable cost [a]	Reasonable cost [a]	14.58 [b]	14.30 [b]
1976	Negotiated rate [a,7] Reasonable cost	Reasonable cost [a,7]	13.25 [b]	13.00 [b]
1975	Negotiated rate [a]	Negotiated rate [a]	12.44 [b]	10.84 [b]
1974	Negotiated rate [a]	Negotiated rate [a]	10.14 [e]	N.A.
1973	Negotiated rate [a]	Negotiated rate [a]	9.69 [f]	N.A.
Montana				
1977	Reasonable cost	Reasonable cost	20.46 [b]	17.32 [b]
1976	Reasonable cost	Reasonable cost	19.03 [b]	16.12 [b]
1975	Reasonable cost	Reasonable cost	17.48 [b]	14.79 [b]
1974	Reasonable cost	Reasonable cost	10.41 [e]	7.46 [e]
1973	Reasonable cost	Reasonable cost	10.82 [f]	7.59 [f]
Nebraska				
1977	Reasonable cost	Reasonable cost	27.18 [a]	15.66 [a]
1976	Negotiated rate	Negotiated rate	13.93 [a]	9.53 [a]
1975	Negotiated rate [a,8]	Negotiated rate [a,8]	11.18 [d]	8.43 [d]
1974	Negotiated rate [a,8]	Negotiated rate [a,8]	9.69 [e]	6.21 [e]
1973	Negotiated rate [a,8]	Negotiated rate [a,8]	N.A.	N.A.
Nevada				
1977	Actual cost with ceiling [a]	Actual cost with ceiling [a]	28.40 [a]	22.00 [b]
1976	Actual cost with ceiling [a]	Actual cost with ceiling [a]	26.73 [a]	20.00 [b]
1975	Actual cost with ceiling [a]	Actual cost with ceiling [a,9]	23.40 [a]	17.26 [b]

Year	Reimbursement Method		Average Per Diem Cost	
	Skilled-Care Facility	Intermediate-Care Facility	Skilled-Care Facility	Intermediate-Care Facility
Nevada continued				
1974	Fixed rate,[a] actual cost with ceiling	Fixed rate[a]	17.34[e]	10.58[e]
1973	Actual cost[a]	Fixed rate[a]	17.20[f]	9.25[f]
New Hampshire				
1977	Reasonable cost	Fixed cost	36.91[c]	24.43[c]
1976	Reasonable cost	Fixed cost	32.21[c]	19.34[c]
1975	Reasonable cost	Fixed cost	24.65[d]	11.07[d]
1974	Reasonable cost	Fixed cost	20.26[e]	11.07[e]
1973	Reasonable cost	Fixed cost	17.72[f]	N.A.
New Jersey				
1977	Reasonable cost with ceiling	Reasonable cost with ceiling	26.00[c]	22.23[b]
1976	Reasonable cost with ceiling	Reasonable cost with ceiling	24.28[c]	20.39[b]
1975	Reasonable cost with ceiling	Reasonable cost with ceiling	22.77[b]	19.60[b]
1974	Reasonable cost with ceiling	Reasonable cost with ceiling	18.40[e]	18.44[e]
1973	N.A.	N.A.	17.08[f]	N.A.
New Mexico				
1977	Reasonable cost	Reasonable cost	N.A.	N.A.
1976	Reasonable cost	Reasonable cost	N.A.	N.A.
1975	Reasonable cost	Reasonable cost	17.68[d]	12.93[d]
1974	Lowest of: 1. Billed charge 2. Reasonable cost 3. $20.00	Lowest of: 1. Billed charge 2. Reasonable cost 3. $17.03	14.49[e]	9.54[e]
1973	Lowest of: 1. Billed charge 2. Reasonable cost 3. $20.00	Lowest of: 1. Billed charge 2. Reasonable cost 3. $17.03	13.93[f]	8.28[f]
New York				
1977	Reasonable cost	Fee schedule	49.65[c]	31.68[c]
1976	Reasonable cost	Fee schedule	45.61[c]	28.18[c]
1975	Reasonable cost	Fee schedule	N.A.	N.A.
1974	Reasonable cost	Fee schedule	N.A.	N.A.
1973	N.A.	N.A.	N.A.	N.A.

	Reimbursement Method		Average Per Diem Cost	
Year	Skilled-Care Facility	Intermediate-Care Facility	Skilled-Care Facility	Intermediate-Care Facility
North Carolina				
1977	Reasonable cost with ceiling	Reasonable cost not to exceed Medicare	23.30 [c]	22.29 [c]
1976	Reasonable cost with ceiling	Reasonable cost not to exceed Medicare	23.30 [c]	21.25 [c]
1975	Reasonable cost with ceiling	Reasonable cost not to exceed Medicare	18.70 [b]	16.04 [b]
1974	Reasonable cost with ceiling	Reasonable cost not to exceed skilled-care facility	N.A.	N.A.
1973	Reasonable cost with ceiling	N.A.	N.A.	N.A.
North Dakota				
1977	Actual cost	Cost at least 10 percent less than skilled-care facilities	21.77 [c]	14.17 [c]
1976	Actual cost	Cost at least 10 percent less than skilled-care facilities	20.36 [c]	13.19 [c]
1975	Actual cost	Cost at least 10 percent less than skilled-care facility	14.57 [b]	11.30 [b]
1974	Actual cost	Cost at least 10 percent less than skilled-care facility	11.08 [e]	6.94 [e]
1973	N.A.	N.A.	9.03 [f]	N.A.
Ohio				
1977	Fixed rate	Fixed rate	18.12 [c]	14.26 [c]
1976	Reasonable cost with ceiling	Reasonable cost with ceiling	16.31 [c]	13.34 [c]
1975	Reasonable cost with ceiling	Reasonable cost with ceiling	13.28 [d]	10.87 [d]
1974	Reasonable cost with ceiling	Reasonable cost with ceiling	9.81 [e]	8.17 [e]
1973	N.A.	N.A.	15.93 [f]	N.A.
Oklahoma				
1977	Negotiated rate	Negotiated rate	15.33 [b]	13.99 [b]
1976	Negotiated rate	Negotiated rate	15.25 [b]	12.84 [b]

Year	Reimbursement Method		Average Per Diem Cost	
	Skilled-Care Facility	Intermediate-Care Facility	Skilled-Care Facility	Intermediate-Care Facility
Oklahoma continued				
1975	Negotiated rate	Negotiated rate	13.26 [b]	12.46 [b]
1974	Negotiated rate	Negotiated rate	10.41 [e]	9.16 [e]
1973	Negotiated rate	Negotiated rate	9.47 [f]	8.37 [f]
Oregon				
1977	Fixed rate [10]	Fixed rate	15.94 [b]	14.08 [b]
1976	Fixed rate	Fixed rate	14.56 [b]	12.95 [b]
1975	Fixed rate	Fixed rate	12.26 [b]	10.98 [b]
1974	Fixed rate	Fixed rate	10.56 [e]	6.48 [e]
1973	Fixed rate	Fixed rate	9.62 [f]	7.28 [f]
Pennsylvania				
1977	Fixed rate	Fixed rate	26.36 [c]	23.53 [c]
1976	Fixed rate	Fixed rate	25.33 [c]	22.03 [c]
1975	Fixed rate	Fixed rate	20.27 [b]	14.38 [b]
1974	Fixed rate	Fixed rate	N.A.	N.A.
1973	Fixed rate	Fixed rate	16.89 [f]	9.90 [f]
Rhode Island				
1977	Reasonable cost with ceiling	Reasonable cost	26.34 [c]	N.A.
1976	Reasonable cost with ceiling	Reasonable cost	24.77 [c]	N.A.
1975	Reasonable cost with ceiling	Reasonable cost	N.A.	N.A.
1974	Reasonable cost with ceiling	Reasonable cost	N.A.	N.A.
1973	Reasonable cost with ceiling	N.A.	N.A.	N.A.
South Carolina				
1977	Allowable cost	Allowable cost	28.92 [c]	22.52 [c 11]
1976	Allowable cost with ceiling	Fixed $624/month	25.82 [c]	20.46 [c 11]
1975	Allowable cost with ceiling	Fixed $450/month	19.34 [b]	12.93 [b]
1974	Allowable cost with ceiling	Fixed $315/month	13.91 [e]	10.33 [11]
1973	Allowable cost with ceiling	Fixed $265/month	13.47 [f]	8.69 [11]

	Reimbursement Method		Average Per Diem Cost	
Year	Skilled-Care Facility	Intermediate-Care Facility	Skilled-Care Facility	Intermediate-Care Facility
South Dakota				
1977	Reasonable cost	Reasonable cost	17.50 [a]	14.66 [a]
1976	Actual cost with adjusted ceiling [a,12]	Actual cost with adjusted ceiling [a,12]	14.81 [a]	12.50 [a]
1975	Actual cost with adjusted ceiling [a,12]	Actual cost with adjusted ceiling [a,12]	14.34 [a]	12.21 [a]
1974	Actual operating cost with ceiling [a]	Actual operating cost with fixed ceiling [a]	9.25 [e]	7.70 [e]
1973	Actual operating cost with ceiling [a]	Actual operating cost with fixed ceiling [a]	8.33 [f]	6.97 [f]
Tennessee				
1977	Reasonable cost with ceiling	Reasonable cost with ceiling	28.99 [c]	16.01 [c]
1976	Reasonable cost with ceiling	Reasonable cost with ceiling	29.46 [c]	15.37 [c]
1975	Reasonable cost with ceiling	Reasonable cost with ceiling	25.12 [b]	11.80 [b]
1974	Reasonable cost with ceiling	Reasonable cost with ceiling	19.58 [e]	8.09 [e]
1973	Reasonable cost with ceiling	Reasonable cost with ceiling	18.44 [f]	6.36 [f]
Texas				
1977	Fixed rate	Fixed rate	17.88 [b]	15.02 [b]
1976	Fixed rate	Fixed rate	16.79 [b]	14.13 [b]
1975	Fixed rate	Fixed rate	14.30 [b]	11.83 [b]
1974	Fixed rate	Fixed rate	12.84 [e]	9.85 [e]
1973	Fixed rate	Fixed rate	11.75 [f]	8.84 [f]
Utah				
1977	Reasonable cost	Reasonable cost	22.50 [b]	15.81 [b]
1976	Reasonable cost	Reasonable cost	20.50 [b]	14.00 [b]
1975	Reasonable cost	Reasonable cost	17.07 [b]	11.94 [b]
1974	Reasonable cost	Reasonable cost	11.29 [e]	7.60 [e]
1973	Reasonable cost	N.A.	10.88 [f]	8.62 [f]
Vermont				
1977	Reasonable cost	Reasonable cost	25.15 [c]	20.89 [c]
1976	Reasonable cost	Reasonable cost	22.57 [c]	19.44 [c]
1975	Reasonable cost	Reasonable cost	21.11 [d]	17.16 [d]
1974	Reasonable cost	Reasonable cost	17.65 [e]	15.69 [e]
1973	Reasonable cost	Reasonable cost	19.09 [f]	14.36 [f]

Year	Reimbursement Method		Average Per Diem Cost	
	Skilled-Care Facility	Intermediate-Care Facility	Skilled-Care Facility	Intermediate-Care Facility
Virginia				
1977	Reasonable cost	Reasonable cost	35.38 [c]	23.33 [c]
1976	Reasonable cost	Reasonable cost	26.18 [b]	19.06 [b]
1975	Reasonable cost	Reasonable cost	23.51 [b]	17.12 [b]
1974	Reasonable cost	Reasonable cost	20.01 [e]	10.29 [e]
1973	Reasonable cost	Reasonable cost	17.79 [f]	13.16 [f]
Washington				
1977	Reasonable cost	Reasonable cost	19.16 [c]	15.25 [c]
1976	Reasonable cost	Reasonable cost	17.41 [c]	13.35 [c]
1975	Reasonable cost[13]	Reasonable cost[13]	15.44 [b]	12.12 [b]
1974	Fixed rate	Fixed rate	8.96 [e]	4.07 [e]
1973	N.A.	N.A.	8.12 [f]	5.06 [f]
West Virginia				
1977	Reasonable cost	Audited cost with ceiling[14]	27.93 [c]	20.26 [c]
1976	Reasonable cost	Audited cost with ceiling[14]	26.48 [c]	17.56 [c]
1975	Reasonable cost	Audited cost with ceiling[14]	25.94 [b]	13.25 [b]
1974	Reasonable cost	Audited cost with ceiling[14]	N.A.	N.A.
1973	Reasonable cost	Audited cost with ceiling[14]	16.84 [e]	N.A.
Wisconsin				
1977	Reasonable cost	Reasonable cost	21.24 [b]	15.67 [b]
1976	Reasonable cost	Reasonable cost	21.78 [b]	15.62 [b]
1975	Actual cost [a]	Actual cost [a]	15.47 [b]	12.39 [b]
1974	Actual cost [a]	Actual cost [a]	14.94 [e]	7.64 [e]
1973	Actual cost [a]	Actual cost [a]	13.66 [f]	N.A.
Wyoming				
1977	Reasonable cost	Reasonable cost	20.97 [a]	18.87 [a]
1976	Reasonable cost [a]	Reasonable cost [a]	18.95 [a]	17.06 [a]
1975	Reasonable cost [a]	Reasonable cost [a]	16.60 [a]	15.04 [a]
1974	Reasonable cost [a]	Reasonable cost [a]	9.66 [e]	8.48 [e]
1973	Reasonable cost [a]	Reasonable cost [a]	8.57 [f]	8.72 [f]

Note: N.A. means the information was not available.

[1] Considered reasonable-cost method for purposes of analysis.

[2] The reasonable-cost rate began in October 1976 of the fiscal year ending 30 June 1977.

[3] In its Financial Impact Statement (see footnote b), the Florida Medicaid program defines its reimburse-

ment method as the reasonable-cost method. For purposes of the analysis, therefore, Florida uses reasonable cost.

[4] Negotiated rates based on costs. Upper limit on intermediate care in for-profit homes is 85 percent of skilled-care-facility average. Upper limit in nonprofit homes is 75 percent of skilled care facility average.

[5] The reimbursement method used in 1973 was determined by each county within the state. For this reason no one single method was used in Kansas during 1973 to reimburse long-term care.

[6] A reasonable-cost-related method has been used for reimbursement in Louisiana since 1 July 1976. However, as of 26 October 1978 Louisiana has not received DHHS approval for its state plan for Medicaid reimbursement of long-term care. For cost-analysis purposes, use of this reasonable-cost method began with fiscal year 1977.

[7] According to an interview with a Missouri Medicaid official, reasonable-cost reimbursement was implemented effective 1 July 1976 at the start of fiscal year 1977. For cost analysis, the negotiated-rate method is considered as the reimbursement method for fiscal year 1976.

[8] According to an interview with a Nebraska Medicaid administrator, in 1975, 1974, and 1973 the reimbursement method used was the negotiated-rate method, established by individual counties. The reasonable-cost method became effective on 1 July 1976 at the start of fiscal year 1977.

[9] Nevada changed to an actual-cost method of reimbursement effective 1 July 1974 at the start of fiscal year 1975.

[10] Oregon changed to a reasonable-cost-related method effective January 1978, fiscal year 1978.

[11] These per diem figures were calculated by dividing the monthly fixed rate by 30.5.

[12] Actual cost fully reimbursed up to a ceiling. The long-term-care facility then reimbursed a declining percentage on each additional dollar cost above the ceiling.

[13] Reasonable-cost reimbursement began in July 1974 at the start of fiscal year 1975.

[14] Intermediate-care ceiling: $515.00 per month in Title XVIII–approved facility; $380.00 per month in state-licensed facility.

[a] Interviews with Medicaid administrators in the respective state.

[b] U.S., Department of Health, Education, and Welfare, Medical Services Administration, "Financial Impact Statement: Section 249 of PL 92–603." This survey requested state Medicaid programs to report average per diem costs for skilled-care facilities and intermediate-care facilities.

[c] Questionnaire issued for this study requesting state Medicaid programs to report average per diem costs for skilled-care facilities and intermediate-care facilities and to declare whether the states used prospective or retrospective reimbursement in 1977 and 1976.

[d] U.S., Department of Health, Education, and Welfare, Health Care Finance Administration, *State Tables Fiscal Year 1975*, "Medicaid Recipients, Payments, and Services," pp. 14, 136, and 142.

[e] U.S., Department of Health, Education, and Welfare, Social and Rehabilitation Services, *Medicaid Recipient Characteristics—1974*, pp. 53 and 61; *Number of Recipients and Amounts of Payments Under Medicaid—1974*, p. 22.

[f] U.S., Department of Health, Education, and Welfare, Social and Rehabilitation Services, *Medicaid Recipient Characteristics—1973*, pp. 34 and 42; *Number of Recipients and Amounts of Payments under Medicaid—1973*, p. 20.

Appendix C
Prospective and
Retrospective States:
Cost and Utilization
Data for 1975–1977

Skilled Care, 1977

State	Number of Patients per Elderly	Patient Days per Elderly	Average Stay	Per Diem Cost
Prospective States				
Alabama	N.A.	N.A.	N.A.	$21.16
Arkansas	N.A.	N.A.	N.A.	16.00
California	N.A.	N.A.	N.A.	24.81
Colorado	N.A.	N.A.	N.A.	17.27
Connecticut	N.A.	N.A.	N.A.	26.34
Illinois	N.A.	N.A.	N.A.	22.32
Indiana	N.A.	N.A.	N.A.	25.21
Iowa	N.A.	N.A.	N.A.	30.07
Kansas	N.A.	N.A.	N.A.	24.23
Louisiana	N.A.	N.A.	N.A.	21.06
Minnesota	N.A.	N.A.	N.A.	25.83
Mississippi	N.A.	N.A.	N.A.	24.25
New Mexico	N.A.	N.A.	N.A.	N.A.
New York	N.A.	N.A.	N.A.	49.65
North Dakota	N.A.	N.A.	N.A.	21.77
Ohio	N.A.	N.A.	N.A.	18.12
Oklahoma	N.A.	N.A.	N.A.	15.33
South Carolina	N.A.	N.A.	N.A.	28.92
South Dakota	N.A.	N.A.	N.A.	17.50
Tennessee	N.A.	N.A.	N.A.	38.99
Texas	N.A.	N.A.	N.A.	28.99
Washington	N.A.	N.A.	N.A.	19.16
West Virginia	N.A.	N.A.	N.A.	27.93
Wyoming	N.A.	N.A.	N.A.	20.97
Average	N.A.	N.A.	N.A.	23.69
Retrospective States				
Alaska	N.A.	N.A.	N.A.	N.A.
Delaware	N.A.	N.A.	N.A.	25.85

State	Number of Patients per Elderly	Patient Days per Elderly	Average Stay Stay	Per Diem Cost
Hawaii	N.A.	N.A.	N.A.	41.30
Idaho	N.A.	N.A.	N.A.	20.77
Kentucky	N.A.	N.A.	N.A.	31.57
Maine	N.A.	N.A.	N.A.	56.31
Maryland	N.A.	N.A.	N.A.	19.86
Massachusetts	N.A.	N.A.	N.A.	N.A.
Michigan	N.A.	N.A.	N.A.	20.30
Nebraska	N.A.	N.A.	N.A.	27.18
Nevada	N.A.	N.A.	N.A.	28.40
New Hampshire	N.A.	N.A.	N.A.	36.91
New Jersey	N.A.	N.A.	N.A.	26.00
North Carolina	N.A.	N.A.	N.A.	23.30
Oregon	N.A.	N.A.	N.A.	15.94
Pennsylvania	N.A.	N.A.	N.A.	26.36
Rhode Island	N.A.	N.A.	N.A.	26.34
Vermont	N.A.	N.A.	N.A.	25.15
Virginia	N.A.	N.A.	N.A.	35.38
Average	N.A.	N.A.	N.A.	28.64

Note: N.A. means the information was not available.

Skilled Care, 1976

State	Number of Patients per Elderly	Patient Days per Elderly	Average Stay	Per Diem Cost
Prospective States				
Alabama	30.86	7,361	239	$20.00
Arkansas	14.19	2,682	201	16.00
Colorado	N.A.	N.A.	N.A.	16.45
Connecticut	N.A.	N.A.	N.A.	24.85
Illinois	15.03	2,185	145	21.55
Indiana	10.82	N.A.	N.A.	24.15
Iowa	1.07	54	61	23.46
Louisiana	3.74	549	147	17.69
Minnesota	38.10	7,644	251	23.02
New Mexico	0.86	40	47	N.A.
New York	N.A.	N.A.	N.A.	45.61
North Dakota	26.11	6,805	261	20.36

State	Number of Patients per Elderly	Patient Days per Elderly	Average Stay	Per Diem Cost
Ohio	22.66	4,962	222	16.31
Oklahoma	0.08	4	50	15.25
South Carolina	25.61	4,329	169	25.82
Tennessee	1.53	26	23	29.46
Washington	N.A.	N.A.	N.A.	17.41
West Virginia	0.67	67	100	26.48
Wyoming	N.A.	N.A.	N.A.	18.95
Average	13.67	2,824	147.4	22.38
Retrospective States				
Delaware	2.22	294	133	$22.00
Hawaii	38.07	5,857	154	37.36
Idaho	15.95	2,615	164	17.79
Kentucky	14.69	2,161	147	29.37
Maine	3.20	N.A.	N.A.	47.77
Maryland	19.09	3,727	195	18.40
Massachusetts	35.86	6,395	178	N.A.
Michigan	29.95	5,886	197	19.14
Nevada	21.98	4,288	195	26.73
New Hampshire	6.31	526	129	32.21
New Jersey	3.32	344	104	24.28
North Carolina	13.40	1,932	144	23.30
Oregon	2.47	271	110	14.56
Pennsylvania	40.44	7,100	176	25.33
Rhode Island	N.A.	N.A.	N.A.	24.77
Vermont	11.30	1,055	93	22.57
Virginia	1.66	152	92	26.18
Average	16.24	2,840	147.4	25.74

Skilled Care, 1975

State	Number of Patients per Elderly	Patient Days per Elderly	Average Stay Stay	Per Diem Cost
Prospective States				
Alabama	30.20	6,908	235	$15.49
California	45.28	7,691	179	19.81
Colorado	N.A.	N.A.	N.A.	15.23
Connecticut	N.A.	N.A.	N.A.	23.00

State	Number of Patients per Elderly	Patient Days per Elderly	Average Stay	Per Diem Cost
Indiana	9.98	1,528	153	21.42
Minnesota	28.40	5,994	211	18.44
Missouri	5.60	1,241	222	12.44
New Mexico	2.16	39	19	17.68
New York	N.A.	N.A.	N.A.	N.A.
North Dakota	25.00	6,594	264	14.57
Ohio	17.73	4,471	252	13.28
Oregon	2.20	227	104	12.26
South Carolina	24.00	4,086	170	19.34
Washington	43.34	9,418	217	15.44
Wyoming	12.73	3,099	244	16.60
Average	20.55	4,275	189.2	16.79
Retrospective States				
Delaware	3.96	625	158	12.90
Florida	12.54	3,246	259	13.80
Georgia	42.89	9,575	223	14.39
Hawaii	40.54	5,844	144	29.11
Idaho	16.19	2,474	153	17.45
Iowa	0.65	46	88	18.54
Kansas	6.52	1,121	172	14.16
Kentucky	14.37	2,183	152	26.49
Maine	2.20	N.A.	N.A.	N.A.
Maryland	20.11	3,467	172	16.74
Massachusetts	44.45	7,337	165	21.19
Michigan	30.51	6,011	198	18.84
Montana	27.20	5,439	200	17.48
Nevada	22.07	4,273	194	23.40
New Hampshire	7.49	730	97	24.65
New Jersey	3.64	377	104	22.77
North Carolina	14.82	N.A.	N.A.	18.70
Rhode Island	N.A.	N.A.	N.A.	N.A.
South Dakota	20.29	5,283	260	14.34
Tennessee	1.41	33	28	25.12
Vermont	12.23	1,401	115	21.11
Virginia	3.47	172	99	23.51
West Virginia	1.25	92	74	25.94
Wisconsin	36.88	8,165	221	15.47
Average	16.77	3,233	156.0	19.82

Intermediate Care, 1977

State	Number of Patients per Elderly	Patient Days per Elderly	Average Stay	Per Diem Cost
Prospective States				
Alabama	N.A.	N.A.	N.A.	$18.03
Arkansas	N.A.	N.A.	N.A.	11.48
California	N.A.	N.A.	N.A.	19.72
Colorado	N.A.	N.A.	N.A.	16.41
Connecticut	N.A.	N.A.	N.A.	15.16
Illinois	N.A.	N.A.	N.A.	15.63
Indiana	N.A.	N.A.	N.A.	15.27
Iowa	N.A.	N.A.	N.A.	19.60
Kansas	N.A.	N.A.	N.A.	16.10
Kentucky	N.A.	N.A.	N.A.	18.43
Louisiana	N.A.	N.A.	N.A.	12.52
Minnesota	N.A.	N.A.	N.A.	N.A.
Mississippi	N.A.	N.A.	N.A.	21.50
New Hampshire	N.A.	N.A.	N.A.	24.43
New Mexico	N.A.	N.A.	N.A.	N.A.
New York	N.A.	N.A.	N.A.	31.68
North Dakota	N.A.	N.A.	N.A.	14.17
Ohio	N.A.	N.A.	N.A.	14.26
Oklahoma	N.A.	N.A.	N.A.	13.99
South Carolina	N.A.	N.A.	N.A.	22.52
South Dakota	N.A.	N.A.	N.A.	14.66
Tennessee	N.A.	N.A.	N.A.	16.01
Texas	N.A.	N.A.	N.A.	15.02
Washington	N.A.	N.A.	N.A.	15.25
West Virgina	N.A.	N.A.	N.A.	20.26
Wyoming	N.A.	N.A.	N.A.	18.87
Average	N.A.	N.A.	N.A.	17.54
Retrospective States				
Alaska	N.A.	N.A.	N.A.	N.A.
Delaware	N.A.	N.A.	N.A.	25.85
Hawaii	N.A.	N.A.	N.A.	39.05
Idaho	N.A.	N.A.	N.A.	18.09
Maine	N.A.	N.A.	N.A.	22.95
Maryland	N.A.	N.A.	N.A.	17.56
Massachusetts	N.A.	N.A.	N.A.	N.A.
Michigan	N.A.	N.A.	N.A.	18.90
Nebraska	N.A.	N.A.	N.A.	15.66

State	Number of Patients per Elderly	Patient Days per Elderly	Average Stay	Per Diem Cost
Nevada	N.A.	N.A.	N.A.	22.00
New Jersey	N.A.	N.A.	N.A.	22.23
North Carolina	N.A.	N.A.	N.A.	22.29
Oregon	N.A.	N.A.	N.A.	14.08
Pennsylvania	N.A.	N.A.	N.A.	23.53
Rhode Island	N.A.	N.A.	N.A.	N.A.
Vermont	N.A.	N.A.	N.A.	20.89
Virginia	N.A.	N.A.	N.A.	23.33
Average	N.A.	N.A.	N.A.	21.89

Intermediate Care, 1976

State	Number of Patients per Elderly	Patient Days per Elderly	Average Stay	Per Diem Cost
Prospective States				
Alabama	14.50	3,640	251	$17.85
Arkansas	38.87	9.737	251	11.48
Colorado	N.A.	N.A.	N.A.	15.62
Connecticut	N.A.	N.A.	N.A.	14.30
Illinois	40.46	5,980	148	15.37
Indiana	29.14	N.A.	N.A.	14.38
Iowa	41.95	13,179	318	17.75
Kentucky	15.73	2,806	178	17.30
Louisiana	48.00	11,511	240	11.23
Minnesota	46.69	9,620	269	N.A.
New Hampshire	39.11	11,943	306	19.34
New Mexico	18.80	4,612	245	N.A.
New York	N.A.	N.A.	N.A.	28.18
North Dakota	18.60	4,820	259	13.19
Ohio	13.89	3,519	253	13.34
Oklahoma	50.85	13,386	263	12.84
South Carolina	12.20	2,419	198	20.46
Tennessee	33.57	4,994	225	15.37
Washington	N.A.	N.A.	N.A.	13.35
West Virginia	14.80	N.A.	N.A.	17.56
Wyoming	N.A.	N.A.	N.A.	17.06
Average	29.82	7,298	243.1	16.10

State	Number of Patients per Elderly	Patient Days per Elderly	Average Stay	Per Diem Cost
Retrospective States				
Delaware	19.18	4,152	217	18.17
Hawaii	12.80	2,449	191	34.45
Idaho	24.65	6,041	245	16.14
Maine	32.92	N.A.	N.A.	21.80
Maryland	18.05	4,358	241	16.49
Massachusetts	38.19	7,636	200	N.A.
Michigan	22.45	5,087	227	17.62
Nevada	9.94	1,949	196	20.00
New Jersey	25.86	6,657	257	20.39
North Carolina	10.60	1,999	189	21.25
Oregon	32.17	7,386	230	12.95
Pennsylvania	15.98	2,984	187	22.03
Rhode Island	N.A.	N.A.	N.A.	N.A.
Vermont	43.49	10,045	231	19.44
Virginia	23.63	5,857	248	19.06
Average	23.56	5,123	219.9	19.98

Intermediate Care, 1975

State	Number of Patients per Elderly	Patient Days per Elderly	Average Stay	Per Diem Cost
Prospective States				
Alabama	13.61	3,327	244	$13.77
California	3.91	606	150	15.96
Colorado	N.A.	N.A.	N.A.	14.88
Connecticut	N.A.	N.A.	N.A.	13.25
Indiana	29.60	7,197	243	12.57
Minnesota	31.15	7,631	245	13.26
Missouri	5.61	1,280	228	10.84
New Mexico	18.60	4,379	235	12.93
New York	N.A.	N.A.	N.A.	N.A.
North Dakota	18.41	4,710	256	11.30
Ohio	15.32	4,202	274	10.87
Oregon	33.58	7,412	221	10.98
South Carolina	9.90	2,319	234	12.93
Washington	4.93	602	122	12.12
Wyoming	14.36	3,767	262	15.04
Average	16.58	3,953	226.2	12.91

State	Number of Patients per Elderly	Patient Days per Elderly	Average Stay	Per Diem Cost
Retrospective States				
Delaware	15.30	3,900	255	18.41
Florida	1.56	344	221	10.25
Georgia	15.50	3,106	207	13.65
Hawaii	13.68	2,115	155	18.61
Idaho	25.20	6,062	241	15.23
Iowa	35.70	10,209	289	9.62
Kansas	35.19	8,553	243	11.75
Kentucky	11.11	2,399	216	11.57
Maine	30.67	N.A.	N.A.	N.A.
Maryland	16.64	3,688	222	14.53
Massachusetts	24.68	5,608	227	16.30
Michigan	25.22	5,472	217	16.08
Montana	33.37	4,813	144	14.79
Nevada	8.45	1,577	187	17.26
New Hampshire	36.59	9,686	265	11.07
New Jersey	25.30	6,374	252	19.60
North Carolina	8.88	N.A.	N.A.	16.04
Rhode Island	N.A.	N.A.	N.A.	N.A.
South Dakota	40.14	8,195	204	12.21
Tennessee	29.75	5,318	251	11.80
Vermont	41.25	9,644	234	17.16
Virginia	22.69	5,397	240	17.12
West Virginia	8.96	N.A.	N.A.	13.25
Wisconsin	35.01	8,146	233	12.39
Average	23.51	5,530	225.1	14.49

Appendix D
Number of Medicaid
Patients (65 and over)—
Skilled Care and
Intermediate Care

Number of Medicaid Patients (Aged 65 and over)

State	1976[a]	1975[b]	1974[c]	1973[d]
Skilled Care				
Alabama	11,975	11,417	11,701	9,508
Alaska	132	154	213	257
Arkansas	3,930	5,785	5,354	4,111
California	89,351	93,089	116,179	128,520
Colorado	N.A.	N.A.	N.A.	N.A.
Connecticut	N.A.	N.A.	12,699	12,291
Delaware	113	198	289	306
Florida	16,379	16,888	14,634	15,185
Georgia	16,114	18,443	18,284	18,985
Hawaii	2,284	2,311	1,958	1,769
Idaho	1,292	1,279	2,158	2,352
Illinois	17,596	12,761	10,738	11,183
Indiana	5,844	5,298	4,223	3,451
Iowa	393	235	201	182
Kansas	1,415	1,858	1,902	1,987
Kentucky	5,479	5,288	4,928	4,932
Louisiana	1,328	1,168	5,457	8,618
Maine	410	275	704	942
Maryland	6,680	6,838	6,112	6,189
Massachusetts	24,455	29,868	N.A.	N.A.
Michigan	24,975	24,862	27,521	N.A.
Minnesota	16,953	12,498	14,225	12,216
Mississippi	7,490	6,783	6,226	5,623
Missouri	2,758	3,365	N.A.	5,117
Montana	2,277	2,040	1,895	1,605
Nebraska	739	1,107	1,506	1,469
Nevada	1,033	971	837	764
New Hamshire	574	652	434	356
New Jersey	2,611	2,794	14,458	14,401
New Mexico	81	194	287	405

127

State	1976[a]	1975[b]	1974[c]	1973[d]
New York	N.A.	N.A.	N.A.	N.A.
North Carolina	6,873	7,290	N.A.	5,920
North Dakota	1,958	1,825	2,113	2,215
Ohio	24,674	18,902	16,214	9,339
Oklahoma	28	34	500	3,417
Oregon	656	569	529	710
Pennsylvania	56,777	51,670	45,075	31,240
Rhode Island	N.A.	N.A.	N.A.	N.A.
South Carolina	6,146	5,497	5,961	5,955
South Dakota	1,892	1,725	1,778	1,797
Tennessee	693	622	649	811
Texas	9,123	9,593	11,923	13,147
Utah	1,612	1,411	1,649	1,302
Vermont	599	636	872	1,142
Virginia	732	1,471	681	2,960
Washington	N.A.	15,820	16,300	17,320
West Virginia	143	263	N.A.	64
Wisconsin	21,127	18,880	15,635	15,407
Wyoming	N.A.	420	222	240
Intermediate Care				
Alabama	5,625	5,145	5,674	4,968
Alaska	255	277	224	21
Arkansas	10,767	6,991	7,142	9,193
California	7,167	8,031	9,639	12,040
Colorado	N.A.	N.A.	N.A.	N.A.
Connecticut	N.A.	N.A.	N.A.	N.A.
Delaware	978	765	646	312
Florida	4,719	2,103	1,568	1,813
Georgia	8,502	6,666	3,099	2,429
Hawaii	768	780	407	N.A.
Idaho	1,997	1,991	1,350	N.A.
Illinois	47,383	37,874	36,418	42,327
Indiana	15,734	15,716	13,294	12,792
Iowa	15,397	12,996	11,726	9,892
Kansas	10,354	10,028	8,594	8,628
Kentucky	5,866	4,089	2,351	1,036
Louisiana	17,040	22,729	14,026	6,352
Maine	4,214	3,834	3,833	3,381
Maryland	6,319	5,657	5,334	5,015
Massachusetts	26,045	16,584	N.A.	N.A.
Michigan	18,723	20,551	20,191	N.A.

State	1976 [a]	1975 [b]	1974 [c]	1973 [d]
Minnesota	20,777	13,706	17,296	16,090
Mississippi	1,283	6,259	1,361	1,005
Missouri	6,695	3,369	N.A.	N.A.
Montana	1,864	2,503	1,311	1,181
Nebraska	7,541	7,304	6,819	7,137
Nevada	467	372	315	380
New Hampshire	3,559	3,183	2,584	N.A.
New Jersey	20,350	19,402	13,984	N.A.
New Mexico	1,767	1,674	1,443	1,304
New York	N.A.	N.A.	N.A.	N.A.
North Carolina	5,438	4,370	N.A.	N.A.
North Dakota	1,395	1,344	1,046	N.A.
Ohio	15,122	16,333	13,832	7,545
Oklahoma	17,237	19,423	17,118	21,200
Oregon	8,556	8,696	8,115	8,130
Pennsylvania	22,437	24,455	28,452	3,660
Rhode Island	N.A.	N.A.	N.A.	N.A.
South Carolina	2,929	2,267	3,716	3,829
South Dakota	2,718	3,412	2,335	2,271
Tennessee	15,205	13,118	9,852	9,900
Texas	68,100	62,943	59,857	59,316
Utah	1,493	1,379	1,512	1,446
Vermont	2,305	2,145	1,919	1,538
Virginia	10,419	9,621	8,352	6,615
Washington	N.A.	1,800	1,960	2,720
West Virginia	3,168	1,890	N.A.	N.A.
Wisconsin	22,216	17,926	13,035	N.A.
Wyoming	N.A.	474	678	720

[a] Health Care Financing Administration, *Medicaid State Tables Fiscal Year 1976: Recipients, Payments and Services,* HCFA (NCSS) Rept. B–4, table 12, p. 32.

[b] Health Care Financing Administration, *Medical State Tables Fiscal Year 1975: Recipients, Payments, and Services,* HCFA (NCSS) Rept. B–4, table 12, p. 32.

[c] Social and Rehabilitation Services, *Numbers of Recipients and Amounts of Payments under Medicaid 1974,* DHEW Publication, no. (SRS) 77–03153, (NCSS) Rept. B–4 (FY74), table 10, p.35.

[d] Social and Rehabilitation Services, *Numbers of Recipients and Amounts of Payments under Medicaid 1973,* DHEW Publication, no. (SRS) 77–03153, (NCSS) Rept. B–4 (FY73), table 10, p. 33.

Appendix E
Estimated Population, Aged 65 and Over

Estimated Elderly Population
(*in thousands*)

State	1976[a]	1975[b]	1974[c]	1973[d]
Alabama	388	378	365	349
Alaska	9	9	8	8
Arkansas	277	271	264	254
California	2,121	2,056	1,986	1,915
Colorado	218	210	204	201
Connecticut	330	321	314	305
Delaware	51	50	48	47
Florida	1,383	1,347	1,267	1,139
Georgia	443	430	413	392
Hawaii	60	57	53	51
Idaho	81	79	76	73
Illinois	1,171	1,153	1,134	1,123
Indiana	540	531	522	514
Iowa	367	364	360	359
Kansas	289	285	281	278
Kentucky	373	368	364	353
Louisiana	355	346	337	327
Maine	128	125	122	119
Maryland	350	340	333	324
Massachusetts	682	672	661	653
Michigan	834	815	798	788
Minnesota	445	440	432	426
Mississippi	259	253	246	236
Missouri	608	601	591	581
Montana	77	75	73	71
Nebraska	196	194	191	189
Nevada	47	44	41	36
New Hampshire	91	87	86	84
New Jersey	787	767	749	734
New Mexico	94	90	86	79
New York	2,068	2,030	1,998	1,993
North Carolina	513	492	473	448
North Dakota	75	73	72	70

State	1976 [a]	1975 [b]	1974 [c]	1973 [d]
Ohio	1,089	1,066	1,050	1,039
Oklahoma	339	334	328	318
Oregon	266	259	251	242
Pennsylvania	1,404	1,377	1,348	1,319
Rhode Island	116	113	111	108
South Carolina	240	229	219	207
South Dakota	86	85	84	83
Tennessee	453	441	429	410
Texas	1,193	1,158	1,120	1,073
Utah	94	91	88	85
Vermont	53	52	51	49
Virginia	441	424	410	394
Washington	374	365	354	343
West Virginia	214	211	206	201
Wisconsin	523	512	505	495
Wyoming	34	33	32	32

[a] Administration on Aging, *Facts About Older Americans 1977,* DHEW Publication, no. (OHD) 78-20006, table, "Estimated Population Aged 65 and Over, by State: 1976."

[b] Administration on Aging, *Facts About Older Americans 1976,* DHEW Publication, no. (OHD) 77-20006, table, "Estimated Population Aged 65 and Over, by State: 1975."

[c] Administration on Aging, *Facts About Older Americans 1975,* DHEW Publication, no. 75-20006, table, "Estimated Population Aged 65 and Over, by State: 1974."

[d] Administration on Aging, "Statistical Memo Number 12: Unofficial Estimates by State Older Populations, January 1, 1973," in *Abstract of Statistical Information, 1974,* no. 4846-2.12.

Skilled Care
(*in thousands*)

State	1976 [a]	1975 [b]	1974 [c]	1973 [d]
Alabama	2,856	2,611	2,306	2,211
Alaska	18	21	30	48
Arkansas	742	N.A.	1,216	601
California	16,100	15,813	16,518	17,445
Colorado	N.A.	N.A.	N.A.	N.A.
Connecticut	N.A.	N.A.	3,589	3,030
Delaware	15	31	54	83
Florida	3,810	4,372	3,506	3,531
Georgia	3,410	4,117	4,516	4,470
Hawaii	351	333	359	470
Idaho	211	195	445	637
Illinois	2,558	1,920	1,671	1,072
Indiana	N.A.	811	636	N.A.
Iowa	20	16	8	8
Kansas	232	319	394	428
Kentucky	806	803	752	813
Louisiana	195	138	158	1,926
Maine	N.A.	N.A.	N.A.	N.A.
Maryland	1,304	1,178	1,219	1,172
Massachusetts	4,361	4,930	N.A.	N.A.
Michigan	4,909	4,899	5,678	8,722
Minnesota	3,401	2,637	3,327	2,416
Mississippi	1,878	1,684	1,501	1,259
Missouri	530	746	1,005	1,111
Montana	425	407	398	344
Nebraska	126	184	288	N.A.
Nevada	201	188	142	134
New Hampshire	47	63	66	33
New Jersey	271	289	2,251	3,525
New Mexico	3	3	7	35
New York	N.A.	N.A.	N.A.	N.A.

State	1976 [a]	1975 [b]	1974 [c]	1973 [d]
North Carolina	991	N.A.	N.A.	N.A.
North Dakota	510	481	467	555
Ohio	5,403	4,766	4,380	2,121
Oklahoma	1	5	46	280
Oregon	72	59	66	74
Pennsylvania	9,969	N.A.	N.A.	5,073
Rhode Island	N.A.	N.A.	N.A.	N.A.
South Carolina	1,038	935	792	794
South Dakota	454	449	468	475
Tennessee	12	14	23	37
Texas	1,116	1,293	1,736	1,933
Utah	362	317	384	267
Vermont	55	72	140	170
Virginia	67	73	72	129
Washington	N.A.	3,437	3,940	4,417
West Virginia	14	19	N.A.	N.A.
Wisconsin	N.A.	4,180	3,829	3,833
Wyoming	N.A.	102	56	62

[a] Health Care Financing Administration, *Medicaid State Tables Fiscal Year 1976: Recipients, Payments, and Services,* HCFA (NCSS) Rept. B-4, table 53, p. 137.

[b] Health Care Financing Administration, *Medicaid State Tables Fiscal Year 1975: Recipients, Payments, and Services,* HCFA (NCSS) Rept. B-4, table 53, p. 137

[c] Social and Rehabilitation Services, *Medicaid Recipient Characteristics and Units of Selected Medical Services 1974,* DHEW Publication, no. (SRS) 77-03153, (NCSS) Rept. B-4. (FY74), table 25, p. 54.

[d] Social and Rehabilitation Services, *Medicaid Recipient Characteristics and Units of Selected Medical Services 1973,* DHEW Publication, no. (SRS) 76-03153, (NCSS) Rept. B-4 (FY73), table 17, p. 35.

Appendix G
Medicaid Patient Days (Aged 65 and over)— Intermediate Care

Intermediate Care

(*in thousands*)

State	1976[a]	1975[b]	1974[c]	1973[d]
Alabama	1,412	1,257	1,147	968
Alaska	57	57	40	N.A.
Arkansas	2,697	N.A.	1,715	2,156
California	1,111	1,247	1,117	1,112
Colorado	N.A.	N.A.	N.A.	N.A.
Connecticut	N.A.	N.A.	N.A.	N.A.
Delaware	211	195	158	93
Florida	712	464	326	337
Georgia	1,642	1,335	714	578
Hawaii	146	129	72	N.A.
Idaho	489	478	222	4
Illinois	7,003	8,237	8,285	8,877
Indiana	N.A.	3,821	3,424	N.A.
Iowa	4,837	3,716	3,222	1,292
Kansas	2,665	2,437	2,347	2,285
Kentucky	1,046	882	423	86
Louisiana	4,086	3,755	3,391	1,417
Maine	N.A.	N.A.	N.A.	N.A.
Maryland	1,525	1,254	1,292	1,196
Massachusetts	5,208	3,768	N.A.	N.A.
Michigan	4,242	4,459	4,238	N.A.
Minnesota	4,281	3,357	4,501	3,552
Mississippi	299	319	340	78
Missouri	1,525	769	N.A.	N.A.
Montana	373	360	274	236
Nebraska	2,130	2,084	1,975	N.A.
Nevada	91	69	54	71
New Hampshire	1,086	842	695	N.A.
New Jersey	5,239	4,889	1,767	N.A.
New Mexico	433	394	352	289
New York	N.A.	N.A.	N.A.	N.A.

State	1976 [a]	1975 [b]	1974 [c]	1973 [d]
North Carolina	1,025	N.A.	N.A.	N.A.
North Dakota	361	343	149	N.A.
Ohio	3,832	4,480	3,733	N.A.
Oklahoma	4,538	4,453	4,474	4,244
Oregon	1,964	1,919	1,858	1,051
Pennsylvania	4,190	N.A.	N.A.	434
Rhode Island	N.A.	N.A.	N.A.	N.A.
South Carolina	580	531	485	502
South Dakota	712	696	649	611
Tennessee	2,262	2,345	2,720	2,536
Texas	25,435	22,137	14,889	14,475
Utah	373	317	391	310
Vermont	532	501	431	338
Virginia	2,583	2,288	2,014	1,413
Washington	N.A.	220	483	500
West Virginia	N.A.	N.A.	N.A.	N.A.
Wisconsin	5,009	4,171	2,613	5,397
Wyoming	N.A.	124	182	209

[a] Health Care Financing Administration, *Medicaid State Tables Fiscal Year 1976: Recipients, Payments, and Services,* HCFA (NCSS) Rept. B–4, table 57, p. 143.

[b] Health Care Financing Administration, *Medicaid State Tables Fiscal Year 1975: Recipients, Payments, and Services,* HCFA (NCSS) Rept. B–4, table 57, p. 143.

[c] Social and Rehabilitation Services, *Medicaid Recipient Characteristics and Units of Selected Medical Services 1974,* DHEW Publication, no. (SRS) 77–03153, (NCSS) Rept. B-4 (FY74), table 31, p. 62.

[d] Social and rehabilitation Services, *Medicaid Recipient Characteristics and Units of Selected Medical Services 1973,* DHEW Publication, no. (SRS) 76–03153, (NCSS) Rept. B-4 (FY73), table 23, p. 43.

Appendix H
Average Length of Stay: Medicaid Patients— Skilled Care and Intermediate Care

Average Length of Stay of Medicaid Patients (Aged 65 and over)— Skilled Care

State	1976 [a]	1975 [b]	1974 [c]	1973 [d]
Alabama	239	235	197	233
Alaska	144	142	144	189
Arkansas	201	N.A.	227	146
California	184	179	144	136
Colorado	N.A.	N.A.	N.A.	N.A.
Connecticut	N.A.	N.A.	283	247
Delaware	133	158	190	273
Florida	233	259	240	233
Georgia	212	223	247	235
Hawaii	154	144	184	266
Idaho	164	153	207	271
Illinois	145	151	156	96
Indiana	N.A.	153	151	N.A.
Iowa	61	88	44	48
Kansas	164	172	207	216
Kentucky	147	152	155	165
Louisiana	147	119	29	224
Maine	N.A.	N.A.	N.A.	N.A.
Maryland	195	172	199	189
Massachusetts	178	165	N.A.	N.A.
Michigan	197	198	206	243
Minnesota	251	211	234	198
Mississippi	251	248	241	224
Missouri	192	222	235	217
Montana	187	200	210	215
Nebraska	171	166	192	N.A.
Nevada	195	194	170	176
New Hampshire	129	97	154	95
New Jersey	104	104	156	245
New Mexico	47	19	25	88

State	1976[a]	1975[b]	1974[c]	1973[d]
New York	N.A.	N.A.	N.A.	N.A.
North Carolina	144	N.A.	N.A.	N.A.
North Dakota	261	264	221	251
Ohio	222	252	270	227
Oklahoma	50	154	94	82
Oregon	110	104	126	105
Pennsylvania	176	N.A.	N.A.	162
Rhode Island	N.A.	N.A.	N.A.	N.A.
South Carolina	169	170	133	133
South Dakota	240	260	264	265
Tennessee	23	28	37	46
Texas	122	135	146	147
Utah	225	225	233	215
Vermont	93	115	161	149
Virginia	92	99	107	54
Washington	N.A.	217	242	255
West Virginia	100	74	N.A.	N.A.
Wisconsin	N.A.	221	245	249
Wyoming	N.A.	244	253	254

[a] Health Care Financing Administration, *Medicaid State Tables Fiscal Year 1976: Recipients, Payments, and Services,* HCFA (NCSS) Rept. B–4, table 53, p. 137.

[b] Health Care Financing Administration, *Medicaid State Tables Fiscal Year 1975: Recipients, Payments, and Services,* HCFA (NCSS) Rept. B–4, table 57, p. 137.

[c] Social and Rehabilitation Services, *Medicaid Recipient Characteristics and Units of Selected Medical Services 1974,* DHEW Publication, no. (SRS) 77–03153, (NCSS) Rept. B–4 (FY74), table 25, p. 54.

[d] Social and Rehabilitation Services, *Medicaid Recipient Characteristics and Units of Selected Medical Services 1973,* DHEW Publication, no. (SRS) 76–03153, (NCSS) Rept. B–4 (FY73), table 17, p. 35.

Average Length of Stay of Medicaid Patients (Aged 65 and over)— Intermediate Care

State	1976[a]	1975[b]	1974[c]	1973[d]
Alabama	251	244	202	194
Alaska	227	208	181	27
Arkansas	251	N.A.	234	246
California	157	150	117	88
Colorado	N.A.	N.A.	N.A.	N.A.
Connecticut	N.A.	N.A.	N.A.	N.A.

State	1976[a]	1975[b]	1974[c]	1973[d]
Delaware	217	255	245	304
Florida	151	221	208	185
Georgia	193	207	228	254
Hawaii	191	155	178	N.A.
Idaho	245	241	160	331
Illinois	148	217	228	215
Indiana	N.A.	243	258	N.A.
Iowa	318	289	275	131
Kansas	256	243	273	268
Kentucky	178	216	180	83
Louisiana	240	165	241	225
Maine	N.A.	N.A.	N.A.	N.A.
Maryland	241	222	242	237
Massachusetts	200	227	N.A.	N.A.
Michigan	227	217	210	N.A.
Minnesota	269	245	250	213
Mississippi	233	254	250	78
Missouri	228	228	N.A.	N.A.
Montana	201	144	209	193
Nebraska	282	285	289	N.A.
Nevada	196	187	172	187
New Hampshire	306	265	269	N.A.
New Jersey	257	252	126	N.A.
New Mexico	245	235	244	226
New York	N.A.	N.A.	N.A.	N.A.
North Carolina	189	N.A.	N.A.	N.A.
North Dakota	259	256	143	N.A.
Ohio	253	274	270	N.A.
Oklahoma	263	229	261	213
Oregon	230	221	229	111
Pennsylvania	187	N.A.	N.A.	117
Rhode Island	N.A.	N.A.	N.A.	N.A.
South Carolina	198	234	130	137
South Dakota	262	204	278	268
Tennessee	225	251	274	268
Texas	373	352	248	242
Utah	250	230	259	247
Vermont	231	234	225	214
Virginia	248	240	239	218
Washington	N.A.	122	247	171

State	1976[a]	1975[b]	1974[c]	1973[d]
West Virginia	N.A.	N.A.	N.A.	N.A.
Wisconsin	225	233	188	284
Wyoming	N.A.	262	268	265

[a] Health Care Financing Administration, *Medicaid State Tables Fiscal Year 1976: Recipients, Payments, and Services,* HCFA (NCSS) Rept. B-4, table 57, p. 143.

[b] Health Care Financing Administration, *Medicaid State Tables Fiscal Year 1975: Recipients, Payments, and Services,* HCFA (NCSS) Rept. B-4, table 57, p. 143.

[c] Social and Rehabilitation Services, *Medicaid Recipient Characteristics and Units of Selected Medical Services 1974,* DHEW Publication, no. (SRS) 77-03153, (NCSS) Rept. B-4 (FY74).

[d] Social and Rehabilitation Services, *Medicaid Recipient Characteristics and Units of Selected Medical Services 1973,* DHEW Publication, no. (SRS) 76-03153, (NCSS) Rept. B-4 (FY73), table 23, p. 43.

Appendix I
Reimbursement
Methods: Utilization
and Cost Index

Skilled Care, 1977

State	Medicaid Patients per 1,000 Elderly	Medicaid Patient Days per 1,000 Elderly	Medicaid Average Stay	Medicaid Per Diem Cost
Reasonable-Cost-Related Method				
Average of four Reasonable-Cost-Related Variations	N.A.	N.A.	N.A.	$26.05
		Reasonable Cost		
Alaska	N.A.	N.A.	N.A.	N.A.
Delaware	N.A.	N.A.	N.A.	25.85
Florida	N.A.	N.A.	N.A.	15.50
Georgia	N.A.	N.A.	N.A.	15.00
Hawaii	N.A.	N.A.	N.A.	41.30
Idaho	N.A.	N.A.	N.A.	20.77
Iowa	N.A.	N.A.	N.A.	30.07
Kansas	N.A.	N.A.	N.A.	24.23
Kentucky	N.A.	N.A.	N.A.	31.57
Louisiana	N.A.	N.A.	N.A.	21.06
Maine	N.A.	N.A.	N.A.	56.31
Massachusetts	N.A.	N.A.	N.A.	N.A.
Minnesota	N.A.	N.A.	N.A.	25.83
Mississippi	N.A.	N.A.	N.A.	24.25
Missouri	N.A.	N.A.	N.A.	14.58
Montana	N.A.	N.A.	N.A.	20.46
Nebraska	N.A.	N.A.	N.A.	27.18
New Hampshire	N.A.	N.A.	N.A.	36.91
New Mexico	N.A.	N.A.	N.A.	N.A.
New York	N.A.	N.A.	N.A.	49.65
South Carolina	N.A.	N.A.	N.A.	28.92
South Dakota	N.A.	N.A.	N.A.	17.50
Utah	N.A.	N.A.	N.A.	22.50
Vermont	N.A.	N.A.	N.A.	25.15
Virginia	N.A.	N.A.	N.A.	35.38

State	Medicaid Patients per 1,000 Elderly	Medicaid Patient Days per 1,000 Elderly	Medicaid Average Stay	Medicaid Per Diem Cost
Washington	N.A.	N.A.	N.A.	19.16
West Virginia	N.A.	N.A.	N.A.	27.93
Wisconsin	N.A.	N.A.	N.A.	21.24
Wyoming	N.A.	N.A.	20.97	
Average	N.A.	N.A.	N.A.	26.90
Reasonable Cost with Ceiling				
Alabama	N.A.	N.A.	N.A.	21.16
Connecticut	N.A.	N.A.	N.A.	26.34
New Jersey	N.A.	N.A.	N.A.	26.00
North Carolina	N.A.	N.A.	N.A.	23.30
Rhode Island	N.A.	N.A.	N.A.	26.34
Tennessee	N.A.	N.A.	N.A.	28.99
Average	N.A.	N.A.	N.A.	25.36
Actual Cost				
Colorado	N.A.	N.A.	N.A.	17.27
Indiana	N.A.	N.A.	N.A.	25.21
Maryland	N.A.	N.A.	N.A.	19.86
North Dakota	N.A.	N.A.	N.A.	21.77
Average	N.A.	N.A.	N.A.	21.03
Actual Cost with Ceiling				
Nevada	N.A.	N.A.	N.A.	28.40
Average	N.A.	N.A.	N.A.	28.40
Fixed-Rate Method				
Arkansas	N.A.	N.A.	N.A.	16.00
California	N.A.	N.A.	N.A.	24.81
Illinois	N.A.	N.A.	N.A.	22.32
Michigan	N.A.	N.A.	N.A.	20.30
Ohio	N.A.	N.A.	N.A.	18.12
Oregon	N.A.	N.A.	N.A.	26.36
Pennsylvania	N.A.	N.A.	N.A.	15.94
Texas	N.A.	N.A.	N.A.	17.88
Average	N.A.	N.A.	N.A.	20.21
Negotiated-Rate Method				
Oklahoma	N.A.	N.A.	N.A.	15.33
Average	N.A.	N.A.	N.A.	15.33

Note: N.A. means the information was not available.

Skilled Care, 1976

State	Medicaid Patients per 1,000 Elderly	Medicaid Patient Days per 1,000 Elderly	Medicaid Average Stay	Medicaid Per Diem Cost
Reasonable-Cost-Related Method				
Average of Four Reasonable-Cost-Related Variations	16.8	3,167	161	$24.78
Reasonable Cost				
Alaska	14.67	2,105	144	60.95
Florida	11.84	2,755	233	15.01
Georgia	36.37	7,697	212	14.82
Hawaii	38.07	5,857	154	37.36
Idaho	15.95	2,615	164	17.79
Iowa	1.07	54	61	23.46
Kansas	4.90	803	164	15.39
Kentucky	14.69	2,161	147	29.37
Maine	3.20	N.A.	N.A.	47.77
Massachusetts	35.86	6,395	178	N.A.
Minnesota	38.10	7,644	251	23.02
Montana	29.57	5,522	187	19.03
New Hampshire	6.31	526	129	32.21
New Mexico	0.86	40	47	N.A.
New York	N.A.	N.A.	N.A.	45.61
Utah	17.15	3,860	225	20.50
Vermont	11.30	1,055	93	22.57
Virginia	1.66	152	92	26.18
Washington	N.A.	N.A.	N.A.	17.41
West Virginia	0.67	67	100	26.48
Wisconsin	40.40	N.A.	N.A.	21.78
Wyoming	N.A.	N.A	N.A	18.95
Average	16.98	2,900	151	26.78
Reasonable Cost with Ceiling				
Alabama	30.86	7,361	239	20.00
Connecticut	N.A.	N.A.	N.A.	24.85
New Jersey	3.32	344	104	24.28
North Carolina	13.40	1,932	144	23.30
Ohio	22.66	4,962	222	16.31
Rhode Island	N.A.	N.A.	N.A.	24.77
South Carolina	25.61	4,329	169	25.82
Tennessee	1.53	26	23	29.46
Average	16.23	3,159	150	23.60

State	Medicaid Patients per 1,000 Elderly	Medicaid Patient Days per 1,000 Elderly	Medicaid Average Stay	Medicaid Per Diem Cost
Actual Cost				
Colorado	N.A.	N.A.	N.A.	16.45
Delaware	2.22	294	133	22.00
Indiana	10.82	N.A.	N.A.	24.15
Maryland	19.09	3,727	195	18.40
North Dakota	26.11	6,805	261	20.36
Average	14.56	3,609	196	20.27
Actual Cost with Ceiling				
Nevada	21.98	4,288	195	26.73
South Dakota	22.00	5,280	240	14.81
Average	21.99	4,784	217	20.77
Fixed-Rate Method				
Arkansas	14.19	2,682	201	16.00
California	42.13	7,591	184	22.77
Illinois	15.03	2,185	145	21.55
Michigan	29.95	5,886	197	19.14
Mississippi	28.92	7,253	251	15.86
Oregon	2.47	271	110	14.56
Pennsylvania	40.44	7,100	176	25.33
Texas	7.65	935	122	16.79
Average	22.59	4,238	173	19.00
Negotiated-Rate Method				
Louisiana	3.74	549	147	17.69
Missouri	4.54	872	192	13.25
Nebraska	3.77	644	171	13.93
Oklahoma	0.08	4	50	15.25
Average	3.03	517	140	15.03

Skilled Care, 1975

State	Medicaid Patients per 1,000 Elderly	Medicaid Patient Days per 1,000 Elderly	Medicaid Average Stay	Medicaid Per Diem Cost
Reasonable-Cost-Related Method				
Average of Four Reasonable-Cost-Related Variations	17.6	3,547	168	$19.87
Reasonble Cost				
Florida	12.54	3,246	259	$13.80
Georgia	42.89	9,575	223	14.39
Hawaii	40.54	5,844	144	29.11
Idaho	16.19	2,474	153	17.45
Iowa	0.65	46	88	18.54
Kansas	6.52	1,121	172	14.16
Kentucky	14.37	2,183	152	26.49
Maine	2.20	N.A.	N.A.	N.A.
Massachusetts	44.45	7,337	165	21.19
Minnesota	28.40	5,994	211	18.44
Montana	27.20	5,439	200	17.48
New Hampshire	7.49	730	97	24.65
New Mexico	2.16	39	19	17.68
New York	N.A.	N.A.	N.A.	N.A.
Utah	15.51	3,493	225	17.07
Vermont	12.23	1,401	115	21.11
Virginia	3.47	172	99	23.51
Washington	43.34	9,418	217	15.44
West Virginia	1.25	92	74	25.94
Wyoming	12.73	3,099	244	16.60
Average	17.59	3,428	158	19.61
Reasonable Cost with Ceiling				
Alabama	30.20	6,908	235	15.49
New Jersey	3.64	377	104	22.77
North Carolina	14.82	N.A.	N.A.	18.70
Ohio	17.73	4,471	252	13.28
Rhode Island	N.A.	N.A.	N.A.	N.A.
South Carolina	24.00	4,086	170	19.34
Tennessee	1.41	33	28	25.12
Average	15.30	3,175	157	19.12

State	Medicaid Patients per 1,000 Elderly	Medicaid Patient Days per 1,000 Elderly	Medicaid Average Stay	Medicaid Per Diem Cost
Actual Cost				
Alaska	17.11	2,428	142	50.79
Colorado	N.A.	N.A.	N.A.	15.23
Connecticut	N.A.	N.A.	N.A.	23.00
Delaware	3.96	625	158	12.90
Indiana	9.98	1,528	153	21.42
Maryland	20.11	3,467	172	16.74
North Dakota	25.00	6,594	264	14.57
Wisconsin	36.88	8,165	221	15.47
Average	18.84	3,801	185	21.27
Actual Cost with Ceiling				
Nevada	22.07	4,273	194	23.40
South Dakota	20.29	5,283	260	14.34
Average	21.18	4,778	227	18.87
Fixed-Rate Method				
Arkansas	21.35	N.A.	N.A.	16.00
California	45.28	7,691	179	19.81
Illinois	11.07	1,665	151	18.84
Michigan	30.51	6,011	198	18.84
Mississippi	26.81	6,659	248	14.04
Oregon	2.20	227	104	12.26
Pennsylvania	37.52	N.A.	N.A.	20.27
Texas	8.28	1,117	135	14.30
Average	22.88	3,895	169	16.80
Negotiated Method				
Louisiana	3.38	400	119	12.60
Missouri	5.60	1,241	222	12.44
Nebraska	5.71	948	166	11.18
Oklahoma	0.10	15	154	13.26
Average	3.70	651	165	12.37

Skilled Care, 1974

State	Medicaid Patients per 1,000 Elderly	Medicaid Patient Days per 1,000 Elderly	Medicaid Average Stay	Medicaid Per Diem Cost
Reasonable-Cost-Related Method				
Average of Four Reasonable-Cost-Related Variations	16.1	3,296	177	$15.19
Reasonable Cost				
Florida	11.55	2,767	240	10.80
Hawaii	36.94	6,789	184	23.11
Idaho	28.39	5,865	207	10.04
Iowa	0.56	24	44	18.38
Kansas	6.77	1,403	207	8.86
Kentucky	13.54	2,094	155	17.63
Maine	5.77	N.A.	N.A.	N.A.
Massachusetts	N.A.	N.A.	N.A.	N.A.
Minnesota	32.93	7,702	234	10.87
Montana	25.96	5,458	210	10.41
New Hampshire	5.05	774	154	20.26
New Mexico	3.34	81	25	14.49
New York	N.A.	N.A.	N.A.	N.A.
Utah	18.74	4,364	233	11.29
Vermont	17.10	2,757	161	17.65
Virginia	1.66	177	107	20.01
West Virginia	N.A.	N.A.	N.A.	N.A.
Wyoming	6.94	1,757	253	9.66
Average	14.35	3,001	172	14.53
Reasonable Cost with Ceiling				
New Jersey	19.30	3,005	156	18.40
North Carolina	N.A.	N.A.	N.A.	N.A.
Ohio	15.44	4,171	270	9.81
Rhode Island	N.A.	N.A.	N.A.	N.A.
South Carolina	27.22	3,620	133	13.91
Tennessee	1.51	55	37	19.58
Average	15.87	2,713	149	15.43

State	Medicaid Patients per 1,000 Elderly	Medicaid Patient Days per 1,000 Elderly	Medicaid Average Stay	Medicaid Per Diem Cost
Actual Cost				
Alaska	26.63	3,838	144	31.07
Colorado	N.A.	N.A.	N.A.	N.A.
Delaware	6.02	1.141	190	12.82
Indiana	8.09	1,219	151	19.96
Maryland	18.35	3,661	199	15.50
North Dakota	29.35	6,494	221	11.08
Wisconsin	30.96	7,582	245	14.94
Average	19.90	3,989	191	17.56
Actual Cost with Ceiling				
South Dakota	21.17	5,577	264	9.25
Average	21.17	5,577	264	9.25
Fixed-Rate Method				
Arkansas	20.28	4,609	227	9.57
California	58.50	8,317	144	17.81
Connecticut	40.44	11,433	283	15.37
Illinois	9.47	1,473	156	15.50
Michigan	34.49	7,115	206	17.22
Mississippi	25.31	6,103	241	11.80
Nevada	20.41	3,475	170	17.34
Oregon	2.11	266	126	10.56
Pennsylvania	33.44	N.A.	N.A.	N.A.
Texas	10.65	1,550	146	12.84
Washington	46.05	11,129	242	8.96
Average	27.38	5,547	194	13.70
Negotiated-Rate Method				
Louisiana	16.19	469	29	8.94
Missouri	N.A.	1,700	235	10.14
Nebraska	7.88	1,511	192	9.69
Oklahoma	1.52	141	94	10.41
Average	8.53	955	137	9.80

Skilled Care, 1973

State	Medicaid Patients per 1,000 Elderly	Medicaid Patient Days per 1,000 Elderly	Medicaid Average Stay	Medicaid Per Diem Cost
Reasonable-Cost-Related Method				
Average of Four Reasonable-Cost-Related Variations	12.5	2,650	163	$14.52
Reasonable Cost				
Iowa	0.51	24	48	19.12
Kentucky	13.97	2,305	165	16.72
Maine	7.92	N.A.	N.A.	N.A.
Massachusetts	N.A.	N.A.	N.A.	N.A.
Montana	22.61	4,857	215	10.82
New Hampshire	4.24	401	95	17.72
New Mexico	5.13	448	88	13.93
Utah	15.32	3,146	215	10.88
Vermont	23.31	3,482	149	19.09
Virginia	7.51	328	54	17.79
West Virginia	0.32	N.A.	N.A.	16.84
Wyoming	7.50	1,952	254	8.57
Average	9.85	1,883	142	15.15
Reasonable Cost with Ceiling				
North Carolina	13.21	N.A.	N.A.	N.A.
Rhode Island	N.A.	N.A.	N.A.	N.A.
South Carolina	28.77	3,838	133	13.47
	1.98	90	46	18.44
Average	14.65	1,964	89	15.96
Actual Cost				
Colorado	N.A.	N.A.	N.A.	N.A.
Delaware	6.51	1,776	273	12.79
Indiana	6.71	N.A.	N.A.	N.A.
Maryland	19.10	3,619	189	14.10
Wisconsin	31.13	7,744	249	13.66
Average	15.86	4,380	237	13.52
Actual Cost with Ceiling				
South Dakota	21.65	5,729	265	8.33
Average	21.65	5,729	265	8.33

State	Medicaid Patients per 1,000 Elderly	Medicaid Patient Days per 1,000 Elderly	Medicaid Average Stay	Medicaid Per Diem Cost
Fixed-Rate Method				
Arkansas	16.19	2,368	146	8.98
California	67.11	9,109	136	16.78
Connecticut	40.30	9,934	247	15.65
Michigan	N.A.	11,069	243	N.A.
Mississippi	23.83	5,338	224	10.21
Nevada	21.22	3,738	176	17.20
Oregon	2.93	308	105	9.62
Pennsylvania	23.68	3,846	162	16.89
Texas	12.25	1,802	147	11.75
Average	25.94	5,279	176	13.39
Negotiated-Rate Method				
Louisiana	26.35	5,892	224	9.11
Missouri	8.81	1,913	217	9.69
Nebraska	7.77	N.A.	N.A.	N.A.
Oklahoma	10.75	883	82	9.47
Average	13.42	2,896	174	9.42

Intermediate Care, 1977

State	Medicaid Patients per 1,000 Elderly	Medicaid Patient Days per 1,000 Elderly	Medicaid Average Stay	Medicaid Per Diem Cost
Reasonable-Cost-Related Method				
Average of Four Reasonable-Cost-Variations	N.A.	N.A.	N.A.	$17.94
Reasonable Cost				
Delaware	N.A.	N.A.	N.A.	25.85
Florida	N.A.	N.A.	N.A.	11.62
Georgia	N.A.	N.A.	N.A.	14.10
Idaho	N.A.	N.A.	N.A.	18.09
Iowa	N.A.	N.A.	N.A.	19.60
Kansas	N.A.	N.A.	N.A.	16.10
Louisiana	N.A.	N.A.	N.A.	12.52
Maine	N.A.	N.A.	N.A.	22.95
Massachusetts	N.A.	N.A.	N.A.	N.A.
Minnesota	N.A.	N.A.	N.A.	N.A.
Mississippi	N.A.	N.A.	N.A.	21.60
Missouri	N.A.	N.A.	N.A.	14.30
Montana	N.A.	N.A.	N.A.	17.32
Nebraska	N.A.	N.A.	N.A.	15.66
New Mexico	N.A.	N.A.	N.A.	N.A.
Rhode Island	N.A.	N.A.	N.A.	N.A.
South Carolina	N.A.	N.A.	N.A.	22.52
South Dakota	N.A.	N.A.	N.A.	14.66
Utah	N.A.	N.A.	N.A.	15.81
Vermont	N.A.	N.A.	N.A.	20.89
Virginia	N.A.	N.A.	N.A.	23.33
Washington	N.A.	N.A.	N.A.	15.25
Wisconsin	N.A.	N.A.	N.A.	15.67
Wyoming	N.A.	N.A.	N.A.	18.87
Average	N.A.	N.A.	N.A.	17.83
Reasonable Cost with Ceiling				
Alabama	N.A.	N.A.	N.A.	18.03
Alaska	N.A.	N.A.	N.A.	N.A.
Connecticut	N.A.	N.A.	N.A.	15.16
New Jersey	N.A.	N.A.	N.A.	22.23
North Carolina	N.A.	N.A.	N.A.	22.29
Tennessee	N.A.	N.A.	N.A.	16.01
Average	N.A.	N.A.	N.A.	18.74

State	Medicaid Patients per 1,000 Elderly	Medicaid Patient Days per 1,000 Elderly	Medicaid Average Stay	Medicaid Per Diem Cost
Actual Cost				
Colorado	N.A.	N.A.	N.A.	16.41
Indiana	N.A.	N.A.	N.A.	15.27
Maryland	N.A.	N.A.	N.A.	17.56
Average	N.A.	N.A.	N.A.	16.41
Actual Cost with Ceiling				
Nevada	N.A.	N.A.	N.A.	22.00
North Dakota	N.A.	N.A.	N.A.	14.17
West Virginia	N.A.	N.A.	N.A.	20.26
Average	N.A.	N.A.	N.A.	18.81
Fixed-Rate Method				
Arkansas	N.A.	N.A.	N.A.	11.48
California	N.A.	N.A.	N.A.	19.72
Illinois	N.A.	N.A.	N.A.	15.63
Kentucky	N.A.	N.A.	N.A.	18.43
Michigan	N.A.	N.A.	N.A.	18.90
New Hampshire	N.A.	N.A.	N.A.	24.43
Ohio	N.A.	N.A.	N.A.	14.26
Oregon	N.A.	N.A.	N.A.	14.08
Pennsylvania	N.A.	N.A.	N.A.	23.53
Texas	N.A.	N.A.	N.A.	15.02
Average	N.A.	N.A.	N.A.	17.55
Negotiated-Rate Method				
Hawaii	N.A.	N.A.	N.A.	39.05
Oklahoma	N.A.	N.A.	N.A.	13.99
Average	N.A.	N.A.	N.A.	26.52

Intermediate Care, 1976

State	Medicaid Patients per 1,000 Elderly	Medicaid Patient Days per 1,000 Elderly	Medicaid Average Stay	Medicaid Per Diem Cost
Reasonable-Cost-Related Method				
Average of Four Reasonable-Cost-Variations	25.2	5,819	234	$17.09
Reasonable Cost				
Florida	3.41	515	151	11.62
Georgia	19.19	3,706	193	13.96
Idaho	24.65	6,041	245	16.14
Iowa	41.95	13,179	318	17.75
Kansas	35.83	9,224	256	12.01
Maine	32.92	N.A.	N.A.	21.80
Massachusetts	38.19	7,636	200	N.A.
Minnesota	46.69	9,620	269	N.A.
Montana	24.21	4,856	201	16.12
New Mexico	18.80	4,612	245	N.A.
Rhode Island	N.A.	N.A.	N.A.	N.A.
Utah	15.88	3,972	250	14.00
Vermont	43.49	10,045	231	19.44
Virginia	23.63	5,857	248	19.06
Washington	N.A.	N.A.	N.A.	13.35
Wisconsin	42.48	9,578	225	15.62
Wyoming	N.A.	N.A.	N.A.	17.06
Average	29.38	6,834	233	16.00
Reasonable Cost with Ceiling				
Alabama	14.50	3,640	251	17.85
Alaska	28.33	6,428	227	40.12
Connecticut	N.A.	N.A.	N.A.	14.30
New Jersey	25.86	6,657	257	20.39
North Carolina	10.60	1,999	189	21.25
Ohio	13.89	3,519	253	13.34
Tennessee	33.57	4,994	225	15.37
Average	21.12	4,539	233	20.37
Actual Cost				
Colorado	N.A.	N.A.	N.A.	15.62
Delaware	19.18	4,152	217	18.17
Indiana	29.14	N.A.	N.A.	14.38
Maryland	18.05	4,358	241	16.49
Average	22.12	4,255	229	16.17

State	Medicaid Patients per 1,000 Elderly	Medicaid Patient Days per 1,000 Elderly	Medicaid Average Stay	Medicaid Per Diem Cost
Actual Cost with Ceiling				
Nevada	9.94	1,949	196	20.00
North Dakota	18.60	4,820	259	13.19
South Dakota	31.60	8,281	262	12.50
West Virginia	14.80	N.A.	N.A.	17.56
Average	18.74	5,017	239	15.81
Fixed-Rate Method				
Arkansas	38.87	9,737	251	11.48
California	3.38	523	157	17.64
Illinois	40.46	5,980	148	15.37
Kentucky	15.73	2,806	178	17.30
Michigan	22.45	5,087	227	17.62
Mississippi	4.95	1,155	233	12.90
New Hampshire	39.11	11,943	306	19.34
Oregon	32.17	7,386	230	12.95
Pennsylvania	15.98	2,984	187	22.03
South Carolina	12.20	2,419	198	20.46
Texas	57.08	21,320	373	14.13
Average	25.67	6,486	226	16.48
Negotiated-Rate Method				
Hawaii	12.80	2,449	191	34.45
Louisiana	48.00	11,511	240	11.23
Missouri	11.01	2,508	228	13.00
Nebraska	38.47	10,867	282	9.53
Oklahoma	50.85	13,386	263	12.84
Average	32.23	8,145	240	16.21

Intermediate Care, 1975

State	Medicaid Patients per 1,000 Elderly	Medicaid Patient Days per 1,000 Elderly	Medicaid Average Stay	Medicaid Per Diem Cost
Reasonable-Cost-Related Method				
Average of Four Reasonable-Cost-Related Variations	22.0	5,256	230	$14.56
Reasonable Cost				
Florida	1.56	344	221	10.25
Georgia	15.50	3,106	207	13.65
Idaho	25.20	6,062	241	15.23
Iowa	35.70	10,209	289	9.62
Kansas	35.19	8,553	243	11.75
Massachusetts	24.68	5,608	227	16.30
Minnesota	31.15	7,631	245	13.26
Montana	33.37	4,813	144	14.79
New Mexico	18.60	4,379	235	12.93
Rhode Island	N.A.	N.A.	N.A.	N.A.
Utah	15.15	3,488	230	11.94
Vermont	41.25	9,644	234	17.16
Virginia	22.69	5,397	240	17.12
Washington	4.93	602	122	12.12
Wyoming	14.36	3,767	262	15.04
Average	22.81	5,257	224	13.65
Reasonable Cost with Ceiling				
Alabama	13.61	3.327	244	13.77
New Jersey	25.30	6,374	252	19.60
North Carolina	8.88	N.A.	N.A.	16.04
Ohio	15.32	4,202	274	10.87
Tennessee	29.75	5,318	251	11.80
Average	18.57	4,805	255	14.42
Actual Cost				
Colorado	N.A.	N.A.	N.A.	14.88
Connecticut	N.A.	N.A.	N.A.	13.25
Delaware	15.30	3,900	255	18.41
Indiana	29.60	7,197	243	12.57
Maryland	16.64	3,688	222	14.53
Wisconsin	35.01	8,146	233	12.39
Average	24.14	5,733	238	14.34

State	Medicaid Patients per 1,000 Elderly	Medicaid Patient Days per 1,000 Elderly	Medicaid Average Stay	Medicaid Per Diem Cost
Actual Cost with Ceiling				
Alaska	30.78	6,417	208	33.43
Nevada	8.45	1,577	187	17.26
North Dakota	18.41	4,710	256	11.30
South Dakota	40.14	8,195	204	12.21
West Virginia	8.96	N.A.	N.A.	13.25
Average	21.35	5,224	213	17.49
Fixed-Rate Method				
Arkansas	25.80	N.A.	N.A.	11.48
California	3.91	606	150	15.96
Illinois	32.85	7,144	217	16.08
Kentucky	11.11	2,399	216	11.57
Michigan	25.22	5,472	217	16.08
Mississippi	4.98	1,261	254	12.83
New Hampshire	36.59	9,686	265	11.07
Oregon	33.58	7,412	221	10.98
Pennsylvania	17.76	N.A.	N.A.	14.38
South Carolina	9.90	2,319	234	12.93
Texas	54.35	19,116	352	11.83
Average	23.28	6,157	236	13.20
Negotiated-Rate Method				
Hawaii	13.68	2,115	155	18.61
Louisiana	65.69	10,852	165	11.74
Missouri	5.61	1,280	228	10.84
Nebraska	37.65	10,746	285	8.43
Oklahoma	58.15	13,333	229	12.46
Average	36.16	7,665	212	12.42

Intermediate Care, 1974

State	Medicaid Patients per 1,000 Elderly	Medicaid Patient Days per 1,000 Elderly	Medicaid Average Stay	Medicaid Per Diem Cost
Reasonable-Cost-Related Method				
Average of Four Reasonable-Cost-Variations	21.9	5,159	229	$10.04
Reasonable Cost				
Florida	1.24	257	208	7.75
Idaho	17.76	2,924	160	5.27
Iowa	32.57	8,950	275	8.04
Kansas	30.58	8,355	273	5.74
Massachusetts	N.A.	N.A.	N.A.	N.A.
Minnesota	40.04	10,419	250	7.34
Montana	17.96	3,764	209	7.46
New Mexico	16.78	4,099	244	9.54
Rhode Island	N.A.	N.A.	N.A.	N.A.
Utah	17.54	4,450	259	7.60
Vermont	37.63	8,458	225	15.69
Virginia	20.37	4,914	239	10.29
Wyoming	21.19	5,688	268	8.48
Average	23.06	5,662	237	8.47
Reasonable Cost with Ceiling				
New Jersey	18.67	2,359	126	18.44
North Carolina	N.A.	N.A.	N.A.	N.A.
Ohio	13.17	3,556	270	8.17
Tennessee	22.97	6,340	274	8.09
Average	18.27	4,085	223	11.57
Actual Cost				
Colorado	N.A.	N.A.	N.A.	N.A.
Delaware	13.46	3,303	245	11.37
Indiana	25.47	6,559	258	11.60
Maryland	16.02	3,880	242	13.72
Wisconsin	25.81	5,174	188	7.64
Average	20.19	4,729	233	11.08

State	Medicaid Patients per 1,000 Elderly	Medicaid Patient Days per 1,000 Elderly	Medicaid Average Stay	Medicaid Per Diem Cost
Actual Cost with Ceiling				
Alaska	28.00	5,065	181	24.06
North Dakota	14.53	2,076	143	6.94
South Dakota	27.80	7,729	278	7.70
West Virginia	N.A.	N.A.	N.A.	N.A.
Average	23.44	4,957	200	12.90
Fixed-Rate Method				
Arkansas	27.05	6,496	234	7.23
California	4.85	562	117	14.59
Connecticut	N.A.	N.A.	N.A.	N.A.
Illinois	32.11	7,306	228	13.93
Kentucky	6.46	1,163	180	8.38
Michigan	25.30	5,311	210	13.93
Mississippi	5.53	1,385	250	10.58
Nevada	7.68	1,319	172	10.58
New Hampshire	30.05	8,085	269	11.07
Oregon	32.33	7,405	229	6.48
Pennsylvania	21.11	N.A.	N.A.	N.A.
South Carolina	16.97	2,216	130	10.33
Texas	53.44	13,294	248	9.85
Washington	5.54	1,365	247	4.07
Average	20.65	4,659	209	10.09
Negotiated-Rate Method				
Hawaii	7.68	1,369	178	18.15
Louisiana	41.62	10,065	241	8.49
Missouri	N.A.	N.A.	N.A.	N.A.
Nebraska	35.70	10,340	289	6.21
Oklahoma	52.19	13,641	261	9.16
Average	34.30	8,854	242	10.50

Intermediate Care, 1973

State	Medicaid Patients per 1,000 Elderly	Medicaid Patient Days per 1,000 Elderly	Medicaid Average Stay	Medicaid Per Diem Cost
Reasonable-Cost-Related Method				
Average of Four Reasonable-Cost-Related Variations	20.5	4,261	237	$ 8.98
Reasonable Cost				
Iowa	27.55	3,600	131	7.50
Massachusetts	N.A.	N.A.	N.A.	N.A.
Montana	16.63	3,324	193	7.59
New Mexico	16.51	3,660	226	8.28
Vermont	31.39	6,899	214	14.36
Virginia	16.79	3,586	218	13.16
Wyoming	22.50	6,547	265	8.72
Average	21.90	4,603	207	9.94
Reasonable Cost with Ceiling				
Tennessee	24.15	6,186	268	6.36
Average	24.15	6,186	268	6.36
Actual Cost				
Colorado	N.A.	N.A.	N.A.	N.A.
Delaware	6.64	1,995	304	4.54
Maryland	15.48	3,693	237	12.27
Wisconsin	N.A.	10,903	284	N.A.
Average	11.06	1,899	275	8.41
Actual Cost With Ceiling				
South Dakota	27.36	7,366	268	6.97
West Virginia	N.A.	N.A.	N.A.	N.A.
Average	27.36	7,366	268	6.97
Fixed-Rate Method				
Arkansas	36.19	8,490	246	$ 6.82
California	6.29	580	88	10.60
Connecticut	N.A.	N.A.	N.A.	N.A.
Kentucky	2.93	245	83	8.19
Michigan	N.A.	N.A.	N.A.	N.A.
Mississippi	4.26	331	78	6.92
Nevada	10.56	1,982	187	9.25

State	Medicaid Patients per 1,000 Elderly	Medicaid Patient Days per 1,000 Elderly	Medicaid Average Stay	Medicaid Per Diem Cost
Fixed-Rate Method continued				
New Hampshire	N.A.	N.A.	N.A.	N.A.
Oregon	33.60	4,345	111	7.28
Pennsylvania	2.77	329	117	9.90
South Carolina	18.50	2,428	137	8.69
Texas	55.28	13,490	242	8.84
Average	18.93	3,580	143	8.50
Negotiated-Rate Method				
Louisiana	19.43	4,334	225	7.89
Missouri	N.A.	N.A.	N.A.	N.A.
Nebraska	37.76	N.A.	N.A.	N.A.
Oklahoma	66.67	13,348	213	8.37
Average	41.28	8,841	219	8.13

Appendix J
Cost and Utilization
Analysis of Reasonable-
Cost-Related Variations

Four variations of reasonable-cost-related reimbursement were grouped together under the category of the reasonable-cost-related-reimbursement method. These four variations are: reasonable cost, reasonable cost with ceiling, actual cost, and actual cost with ceiling. Each of these variations was given separate codes for computer analysis. These four different methods were grouped two different ways, reasonable cost/reasonable cost with ceiling versus actual cost/actual cost with ceiling and reasonable/ actual cost versus reasonable cost with ceiling/actual cost with ceiling, to discover if statistically significant differences existed between these reasonable-cost-related variations.

The difference of means tests were performed between the sets of groupings for the various dependents variables. The null hypothesis was always that no significant differences exist between groupings. In other words, the grouping are not separate populations but subgroups of the population reasonable-cost-related reimbursement. As the tables in this appendix demonstrate, the null hypothesis was almost never rejected at the .10 significance level.

The major conclusion is that reasonable cost, reasonable cost with ceiling, actual cost, and actual cost with ceiling are subgroups of the reasonable-cost-related method and not separate populatons to themselves. These four variations were therefore combined for reasons of comparison with the negotiated-rate and fixed-cost methods for the cost and utilization indexes. The analysis of variance between these three reimbursement methods for the dependent variables is reported in chapter 4 in the section, "Analysis of Reimbursement Methods."

Reasonable Cost versus Actual Cost

The null hypothesis states that reasonable cost and actual cost are not separate populations but subgroups of the reasonable-cost method. The level of significance is .10.

161

Skilled Care

Year	Reasonable Cost	Actual Cost	Level of Significance
Medicaid Patients (Aged 65 and over) per 1,000 Elderly			
1976	16.8	17.0	0.97
1975	17.0	19.4	0.67
1974	14.7	20.1	0.28
1973	10.9	17.0	0.23
Medical Patient Days (Aged 65 and over) per 1,000 Elderly			
1976	2,968	4,079	0.41
1975	3,373	4,046	0.58
1974	2,937	4,216	0.25
1973	1,898	4,718	0.03
Average Length of Stay for Medicaid Patients			
1976	151	205	0.09
1975	159	196	0.18
1974	167	202	0.26
1973	133	244	0.01
Average Per Diem Cost for Medicaid			
1977	$26.61	$22.50	0.34
1976	25.87	20.41	0.20
1975	19.49	20.79	0.63
1974	14.73	16.37	0.51
1973	15.28	12.22	0.17
Average Per Diem–Dollar Cost Increases for Medicaid			
1976–1977	$2.84	$1.28	0.22
1975–1976	3.17	3.47	0.78
1974–1975	5.08	4.52	0.75
1973–1974	0.61	0.90	0.65

Intermediate Care

Year	Reasonable Cost	Actual Cost	Level of Significance
Medicaid Patients (Aged 65 and over) per 1,000 Elderly			
1976	26.9	20.1	0.19
1975	21.7	22.6	0.84
1974	22.0	21.6	0.92
1973	22.2	16.5	0.29

Year	Reasonable Cost	Actual Cost	Level of Significance
Medicaid Patient Days (Aged 65 and over) per 1,000 Elderly			
1976	6,110	4,713	0.37
1975	5,157	5,479	0.77
1974	5,324	4,827	0.69
1973	4,830	3,267	0.29
Average Length of Stay for Medicaid			
1976	233	235	0.93
1975	231	226	0.74
1974	234	219	0.49
1973	216	273	0.06
Average Per Diem Cost for Medicaid			
1977	$18.01	$17.61	0.81
1976	17.53	15.99	0.50
1975	13.85	15.77	0.25
1974	9.14	11.86	0.21
1973	9.42	7.93	0.53
Average Per Diem–Dollar Cost Increases for Medicaid			
1976–1977	$1.46	$1.41	0.92
1975–1976	2.37	1.69	0.41
1974–1975	4.53	4.54	0.99
1973–1974	0.23	3.00	0.10

A level of significance of .10 or less is required to reject the null hypothesis. In almost all tests of the null hypothesis, the observed level of significance is higher than .10. The conclusion is that the reasonable-cost- and actual-cost-reimbursement methods are actually subgroups of the reasonable-cost-reimbursement method and not separate populations.

Cost without Ceilings versus Cost with Ceilings

The null hypothesis states that cost without ceilings and cost with ceilings are not separate populations but subgroups of the reasonable-cost-reimbursement method. The level of significance is .10.

Skilled Care

Year	Cost without Ceilings	Cost with Ceilings	Level of Significance
Medicaid Patients (Aged 65 and over) per 1,000 Elderly			
1976	16.6	17.7	0.84
1975	17.9	16.8	0.84
1974	15.9	16.9	0.86
1973	11.5	16.4	0.37
Medicaid Patient Days (Aged 65 and over) per 1,000 Elderly			
1976	3,007	3,566	0.62
1975	3,522	3,633	0.93
1974	3,298	3,286	0.99
1973	2,507	3,219	0.65
Average Length of Stay for Medicaid Patients			
1976	159	167	0.76
1975	165	178	0.68
1974	178	172	0.86
1973	166	148	0.75
Average Per Diem Cost for Medicaid			
1977	$26.11	$25.79	0.93
1976	25.48	23.03	0.52
1975	20.12	19.06	0.71
1974	15.44	14.19	0.65
1973	14.77	13.41	0.57
Average Per Diem–Dollar Cost Increases for Medicaid			
1976–1977	$3.08	$1.02	0.06
1975–1976	3.58	3.53	0.97
1974–1975	4.96	4.78	0.93
1973–1974	0.65	0.83	0.80

Intermediate Care

Year	Cost without Ceilings	Cost with Ceilings	Level of Significance
Medicaid Patients (Aged 65 and over) per 1,000 Elderly			
1976	28.1	20.2	0.08
1975	23.1	20.0	0.48
1974	22.3	20.9	0.75
1973	19.2	25.8	0.29

Year	Cost without Ceilings	Cost with Ceilings	Level of Significance
Medicaid Patient Days (Aged 65 and over) per 1,000 Elderly			
1976	6,491	4,699	0.16
1975	5,364	5,015	0.76
1974	5,413	4,521	0.48
1973	3,702	6,777	0.08
Average Length of Stay for Medicaid Patients			
1976	232	235	0.85
1975	227	235	0.65
1974	236	212	0.29
1973	230	268	0.35
Average Per Diem Cost for Medicaid			
1977	$17.65	$18.77	0.46
1976	16.03	18.72	0.20
1975	13.86	15.95	0.22
1974	9.16	12.23	0.12
1973	9.55	6.67	0.28
Average Per Diem–Dollar Cost Increases for Medicaid			
1976–1977	$1.89	$1.28	0.40
1975–1976	1.83	3.20	0.09
1974–1975	4.63	4.30	0.80
1973–1974	1.02	1.23	0.92

A level of significance of .10 or less is required to reject the null hypothesis. In almost all tests of the null hypothesis, the observed level of significance is higher than this benchmark .10 level. The major conclusion is that the cost-without-ceilings- and cost-with-ceilings-reimbursement methods are actually subgroups of the reasonable-cost-reimbursement method and not separate populations.

Appendix K
Cost Analysis of
Section 249 by Medical
Services Administration

State Estimates where Per Diem Rate Increases Expected, 1 July 1976 to 30 June 1977

State	Increase in Rate [a] (dollars)	Patient Days (thousands)	Estimated Impact (thousands)
Skilled-Care Facilities			
Region II			
New Jersey	3.00 (29.00)	400	$ 1,200
Region III			
Delaware	2.00 (21.00)	50	100
District of Columbia	3.00 (30.00)	100	300
Pennsylvania	4.00 (29.00)	8,900	35,600
Region IV			
Mississippi	1.50 (19.50)	2,200	3,300
Region V			
Illinois	5.00 (21.00) [b]	3,400	17,000
Region VI			
Oklahoma	2.50 (18.00)	90	200
Region VII			
Missouri	1.50 (16.00)	1,100	1,700
Nebraska	2.00 (14.50)	200	400
Region VIII			
South Dakota	1.50 (14.50)	600	900
Region X			
Washington	2.00 (19.50)	5,900	11,800
Total			72,500
Intermediate-Care Facilities			
Region II			
New Jersey	3.00 (25.00)	6,500	19.500
Region III			
Delaware	2.00 (24.00)	300	600
District of Columbia	10.00 (25.00)	300	3,000
Pennsylvania	2.50 (21.50)	4,000	10,000
Region IV			
Kentucky	5.00 (16.50)	2,000	10,000
Mississippi	2.00 (17.00)	500	1,000
Region V			
Illinois	1.00 (14.50)	10,800	10,800
Region VI			
Oklahoma	3.00 (16.00)	5,800	17,400

State	Increase in Rate[a] (dollars)	Patient Days (thousands)	Estimated Impact (thousands)
Region VII			
Missouri	1.50 (15.50)	2,400	3,600
Nebraska	1.00 (10.00)	700	700
Region VIII			
South Dakota	.50 (11.50)	900	500
Region X			
Washington	3.00 (16.50)	600	1,800
Total			78,900

Source: U.S., Department of Health, Education, and Welfare, Medical Services Administration, *Inflationary Impact Statement—Section 249 of PL 92-603,* table I for skilled-care data; table II for intermediate-care data.

[a] State estimate of reimbursement rate that would occur based on requirements in draft regulation. The increase is the difference between such rate and the rate that probably would be in effect in the absence of Section 249.

[b] Estimate based on comparison of current average reimbursement rate to average rates paid in contiguous states.

Selected Bibliography

AFL-CIO. *America's Nursing Homes—Profit in Misery*. Washington, D.C., 1977.

Anderson, Nancy, and Hopkins, Holmberg. "Implication of Ownership for Nursing Home Care." *Medical Care* 6(July-August 1968):300–07.

Anderson, Nancy, and Lana Stone. "Nursing Homes: Research and Public Policy." *Gerontologist* 9(Autumn 1969):214–18.

Applied Management Sciences. "Report on Systems of Reimbursement for Long-Term Care," vols. I–III. Silver Spring, Maryland, 1976.

Averrech, Harvey and Leland Johnson. "Behavior of the Firm under Regulatory Constraint." *American Economic Review* 52(December 1962): 1052–69.

Blalock, Hubert. *Social Statistics*. New York: McGraw-Hill, 1960.

Buchanan, Robert. "Public Policy and Long-Term Care." Masters thesis, University of Virginia, 1976.

Business Week. "Nursing the Nursing Homes Back to Health." December 5, 1977:66–70.

———. *"Business Week*'s Corporate Scoreboard." 9 March 1974.

———. *"Business Week*'s Corporate Scoreboard." 24 March 1975.

———. *"Business Week*'s Corporate Scoreboard." 22 March 1976.

———. *"Business Week*'s Corporate Scoreboard." 21 March 1977.

———. *"Business Week*'s Corporate Scoreboard." 20 March 1978.

Commerce Clearing House. *Medicare and Medicaid Guide*. Chicago.

Dye, Thomas. *Understanding Public Policy*. Englewood Cliffs, N.J.: Prentice-Hall, 1978.

Frank, Kenneth. "Government Support of Nursing-Home Care." *New England Journal of Medicine* 257(September 1972):538–45.

Fraundorf, Kenneth. "Competition and Public Policy in the Nursing-Home Industry." *Journal of Economic Issues* 11(September 1977):601–34.

Gaynes, Neil. "A Logic to Long-Term Care." *Gerontologist* 13(Autumn 1973):277–81.

Hermelin, William. Administrator, Government Services, American Health Care Association. Interview, July, 1978.

Inglehart, John. "Government Searching for a More Cost Efficient Way to Pay for Hospitals." *National Journal* 8(25 December 1976):1822–29.

Isack, Arthur. "Federal Government Involvement in Training Medical Director of Long-Term-Care Facilities." *Journal of the American Geriatrics Society* 21:261–63.

Iverson, Gudmund, and Norpoth, Helmut. *Analysis of Variance*. Beverly Hills: Sage Publications, 1976.

Labovitz, Sanford. "Criteria for Selecting a Significance Level: A Note of the Sacredness of .05." *American Sociologist* 3-4(August 1968):220–222.

Levey, Samuel, et al. "An Appraisal of Nursing Home Care." *Journal of Gerontology* 28(February 1973):222–28.

Levin, Jack. *Elementary Statistics in Social Research.* New York: Harper and Row, 1973.

Mendelson, Mary. *Tender Loving Greed.* New York: Alfred A. Knopf, 1974.

Morrison, Denton, and Ramon, Henkel. "Significance Tests Reconsidered." *American Sociologist* 4(May 1969):131–40.

Nauen, Richard. "A Method for Planning for the Care of Long-Term Patients." *American Journal of Public Health* 58(November 1968): 2111–19.

Penchansky, Roy, and Leon Taubenlaus. "Institutional Factors Affecting the Quality of Care in Nursing Homes." *Geriatrics* 20(July 1965):591–98.

Phillips, John. *Statistical Thinking.* San Francisco: W.H. Freeman, 1973.

Redford, Emmett. *Democracy in the Administrative State.* New York: Oxford University Press, 1969.

Ripley, Randall, and Grace Franklin. *Congress, The Bureaucracy, and Public Policy.* Homewood, Ill.: Dorsey Press, 1976.

Roven, Will. "The Changing Environment of the 1970s." *Canadian Hospital* 49(January 1972):48–50.

Ruchlin, Hirsch, Samuel Levey, and Charlotte Muller. "The Long-Term Care Marketplace." *Medical Care* 13:979–91.

Schor, Irving. "Fitting Long-Term Care to the Patient's Need." *Geriatrics* 29(February 1974):163–64.

Shanas, Ethel. "Factors Affecting the Care of the Patient." *Journal of the American Geriatrics Society* 21(September 1973):394–97.

Tannenbaum, Jeffrey. "Medical Squeeze." *Wall Street Journal,* 21 June 1977.

Traska, Marta. "Proprietary Chains Operated 20% More Beds During 1977." *Modern Health Care* 8(June 1978):38, 42–43.

Truman, David. *The Government Process.* New York: Alfred A. Knopf, 1951.

U.S. Congress, Senate, Committee on Finance. *Social Security Amendments of 1972.* Rept. 92-1230. 92nd Cong., 2nd sess., 1972.

U.S. Congress, House of Representatives, Conference Committee. *Social Security Amendments of 1972.* Rept. 92-1605. 92nd Cong., 2nd sess., 1972.

U.S. Congress, Senate, Subcommittee on Long-Term Care. *Nursing Home Care in the United States—Failure in Public Policy.* 93rd Cong., 2nd sess., 1974.

————. *Congressional Record.* 95 Cong., 1st sess., 30 September 1977.

U.S. Congress, House of Representatives, Interstate and Foreign Commerce Committee. *Data on Medicaid Program.* 95 Cong., 1st sess., 1977.

U.S. Congress, Senate, Committee on Finance. *Health Care Cost Containment and Other Proposals.* Committee Print 96-9, 96th Congress, 1st sess., 20 March 1979.

U.S. Department of Health, Education and Welfare. Health Care Finance Administration, Medicaid Bureau. *Data on Medicaid Program: Eligibility, Services, and Expenditures, Fiscal Years 1966-1978.*

————. Social Security Administration. *Principles of Reimbursement for Provider Costs.* DHEW Publication, no. HIM-5, January 1967.

————. Comptroller General of the United States. *Problems in Providing Guidance to the States in Estimating Rates of Payment for Nursing Home Care under Medicaid Program.* 19 April 1972.

————. Social and Rehabilitation Services. *Medicaid Recipient Characteristics and Units of Selected Medicaid Services—1973.* NCSS Rept. B-4 (FY73).

————. Social and Rehabilitation Services. *Number of Recipients and Amounts of payments Under Medicaid—1973.* NCSS Rept. B-4 (FY73).

————. Social and Rehabilitation Services. *Medicaid Recipient Characteristics and Units of Selected Medicaid Services—1974.* NCSS Rept. B-4 (FY74).

————. Social and Rehabilitation Services. *Number of Recipients and Amounts of Payments Under Medicaid—1974.* NCSS Rept. B-4 (FY74).

————. Social Security Administration. *Research and Statistics Note.* 29 November 1974.

————. Health Care Finance Administration. *Medicaid State Tables Fiscal Year 1975: Recipients, Payments, and Services.* NCSS Rept. B-4 (FY75).

————. Social Security Administration. *Research and Statistics Note.* 13 May 1975.

————. Health Care Finance Administration. *Medicaid State Tables Fiscal Year 1976: Recipients, Payments, and Services.* NCSS Rept. B-4 (FY76).

————. Social Security Administration. *Research and Statistics Note.* 22 December 1976.

————. *Federal Register* 43, no. 25 (6 February 1978):4861-64.

Virginia, Department of Health. *1971 Statistical Annual Report.* 1972.

————. *1972 Statistical Annual Report.* 1973.

————. *1973 Statistical Annual Report.* 1974.

―――. *1974 Statistical Annual Report.* 1975.
―――. *1975 Statistical Annual Report.* 1976.
―――. *1976 Statistical Annual Report.* 1977.
Weikel, M. Keith, and Nancy Leamond. "A Decade of Medicaid." *Public Health Reports* 91:303-08.

Index

AFL-CIO Executive Council, 14, 18, 94

AHCA, Inc. v. *Califano*, 84–86

Alabama Nursing Home Association v. *Califano*, 86

American Association of Homes for the Aging, 78

American Health Care Association, 77

Analysis of variance, 49–50

Anta Corporation, Four Seasons Nursing Homes division of, 72, 94–95

Bellmon Amendment, 79–82

Beverly Enterprises, 72

Blue Cross: of New York, 44; of Rhode Island, 43

Byrd, Harry, 99

Califano, Joseph, 84–85, 86

Congressional Budget Office, 99

Cost measures, 53

Curtis, Carl, 77, 78

Davis, Jack, 21

Department of Health and Human Services, 26, 43, 54, 80, 83, 85; guidelines for state Medicaid plans, 83–84

Difference of means, 49

District of Columbia Medicaid program, 32

Fixed-rate reimbursement, 32; analysis of, 63–72

General Accounting Office, 99

Government-policy arena model, 75–76

Group theory, policymaking model, 81–82

Health-care institutions, differentiation, 3

Intermediate-care facility, 4–5

Johns Hopkins reimbursement experiment, 40–41

Kerr-Mills program, 78–79

Lane, Laurence, 78

Levey, Samuel, 27, 39

Long-term-care industry, 13–15; profit motive, 17

Louisiana Medicaid program, 33

Maryland Medicaid program, 41

Medicaid program, 10, 25; health impact, 25–26; Virginia program, 7

Medicaid: reimbursement methods, 30–34; spending, 5–9

Medical Services Administration, 87–89, 99

Medicare spending, 6–7

Michigan Medicaid program, 42

Missouri Medicaid program, 33, 34

Muller, Charlotte, 27, 39

Negotiated rate reimbursement, 32–34; analysis of, 63–72

New Hampshire Medicaid program, 32

New York Medicaid program, 44

Oklahoma Medicaid program, 33

Oklahoma State Nursing Home Association, 33, 82

PL 92-603 (Section 249), 30, 75; Bellmon amendment, 80–82; development, 76–80; inflation impact, 88–89; legislative intent, 83–87

Prospective-rate determination, 41–42; advocates, 41–44; analysis of, 54–62; cost savings, 43–44; criticism, 44–45; recommended system, 100–101

173

About the Author

Robert J. Buchanan received the B.A. in political science from Grinnell College and the M.A. in public administration and the Ph.D. in American government (public affairs) from the University of Virginia. He served as a graduate intern at the Federal Executive Institute for two years while at the University of Virginia. He taught political science and public administration at the University of Nebraska at Omaha. Currently, Professor Buchanan teaches policy analysis, public-sector budgeting, and public financial management at California State College at San Bernardino.